Contents

About the author

Acknowledgements   6

Foreword   7

1 Pain – physical and psychological effects
What have we learned over the centuries?   11
Consciousness and perception of pain   12
What is pain and why do we feel it?   14
Gate Control Theory – how our body reacts   15
The role of the brain and nervous system   17
The diversity of pain   20
Behavioural responses to pain   22
Psychological (emotional and cognitive) aspects of pain   23
The mystery of pain   24
The placebo effect   25
Conclusion   31

2 Pain – types and common causes
Types of pain   35
The nature of pain   38
Treatments   40
Pain caused by cancer   41
Common causes of non-malignant pain   43
Conclusion   83

3 Diagnosis and assessment
Reaction to pain   85
Pain thresholds   88
Tests and investigations   91
Assessing pain   97
Pain clinics   99
Pain assessment tools   101
Barriers to successful pain management   113
Making a complaint   115
Conclusion   115

GW00514659

4 Dealing with the pain – orthodox and self-help treatments
Being realistic   116
Why is it important to treat pain at an early stage?   117
Orthodox or self-help treatments – which routes to choose?   118
Medication   121
How do drugs get into the system?   122
Common pain relievers   124
Non-drug techniques   130
Pain management units – eg 'INPUT'   138
Conclusion   140

5 Stress relief and non-orthodox treatments
What is 'stress'?   141
Helping yourself   146
Learning to relax   149
Complementary treatments to help manage your pain   154
Conclusion   172

6 Looking at your lifestyle
Healthy eating   174
Exercise   178
A better night's sleep   184
Boosting mood   185
Alcohol   187
Smoking   189
Sexual relationships   192
Transport and mobility   194
Holidays   196
Maintaining the good times   198
Conclusion   200

Useful addresses   201

Glossary   211

Bibliography   213

About Age Concern   214

Publications from Age Concern Books   215

**Age Concern Information Line /
Factsheets subscription**   217

Index   218

About the author

Toni Battison is a trained nurse with considerable practical and teaching experience during a career working with older people and carers. She has worked as a District Nursing Sister, a Health Promotion Adviser, a lecturer for a Certificate in Health Education course, and as the manager of a charity. She is now retired from these external roles and works part time on her freelance health education work. Toni has written many publications, including several volumes in Age Concern's series aimed at informal carers. She is an Associate Member of the Guild of Health Writers.

Toni has always been concerned about the need to support carers and patients, to enable them to get the best from local and national services, as she believes that people gain great benefit from being able to help themselves. While working for the Cambridge and Huntingdon Health Authority, she helped create an information centre for patients and visitors at Addenbrooke's Hospital and, with other carers, started the Telephone Information Line for Carers of Elderly People in the Cambridge area. She was joint winner of the Ian Nichol Prize for Health Promotion in 1990 and 1992 for these projects.

Toni lives near Cambridge with her husband, whom she recently nursed back to health following an accident. The couple have three grown-up daughters. She is also the main carer for her mother (now in her late 80s) who lives with her, and she helped her mother care for her father following a series of strokes and epilepsy until he died at home. Her experience of caring for members of her own family has given her a personal perspective that complements her professional role.

Acknowledgements

The author thanks the many people – carers, friends and colleagues – who have contributed valuable help and advice throughout the production of this book. In particular:

- Staff members at the Pain Clinic, Addenbrooke's NHS Trust, Cambridge;
- Dr Eloise Carr of Bournemouth University;
- Ian Semmons, and other members of Action on Pain, for comments, advice, and contributions in the form of case studies;
- Staff members at Age Concern England, especially Richard Holloway, Leonie Farmer and Sue Henning;
- Richenda Milton-Thompson, for editorial input;
- The various people, some of them unknown to me, who have reviewed the draft material and made important suggestions to help improve the text.

In addition I thank all the national organisations that offer information and support to carers in the broadest sense, whose materials have helped to inform and influence my thinking.

Foreword

With chronic pain suffered by one in seven of the UK population, and with an ageing population, the demands on pain services can only increase. So it is critical that those affected can easily access reliable information on self-help. The information contained within this book goes some considerable way towards fulfilling that need.

As somebody who has lived with chronic pain for the last fifteen years, along with the highs and lows that accompany it, I can only encourage you to challenge and try to take control of your pain. At times the pressures on our family have been immense, yet by understanding my pain we have been able to work together to move forward. It has been an interesting and rewarding journey, and if you have doubts about taking this journey yourself, I urge you to go for it! Good luck.

Ian Semmons MBA
Chairman, **Action on Pain**
www.action-on-pain.co.uk

1 Pain – physical and psychological effects

Human bodies experience pain in two ways: as a physical sensation and as a psychological perception. One thing is for sure, we do not like the feeling. The nature of pain is a complex phenomenon and it is one of the most common reasons for visiting a doctor. The need to seek relief from physical discomfort, coupled with the uncertainty and fear of what that pain might represent, are powerful incentives to get help. Historical records and literature leave us in no doubt that, over the centuries and before the discovery of truly effective painkillers, our ancestors must have suffered a great deal of pain. Fortunately, times have changed and much progress has been made in recent years towards understanding and managing pain. Treatments are continually developing, reliable painkilling drugs are readily available in any supermarket, and it is now possible to reassure people with cancer that – whatever the intensity of their pain – it should be well controlled. Yet, despite these advances in knowledge and practice, our understanding of pain is still inadequate. It is difficult to measure, and the way it is perceived by the brain is not yet fully understood. Questions surrounding pain are plentiful, for example:

- How can levels of pain be assessed accurately?
- Does gender or age affect how we feel?
- What is a pain 'threshold'?
- Why is pain apparently tolerated at different intensities?
- Does the doctor or dentist really understand (and believe us) when we try to describe how severe the pain is?

There are no simple answers to these common queries. The concept of pain is influenced by a combination of interacting factors, some of which are fixed, some are variable and others yet again may be subjective only. For example, our inherent body blueprint cannot change, so people are probably programmed to feel pain differently. It also appears that age has a bearing on our ability to cope, and the way we interpret feelings about pain fluctuates depending on how the signal is perceived within the human consciousness. These key issues and many others are covered more fully throughout the book.

This chapter provides basic information about the characteristics of pain and why it occurs. It goes on to describe the role of the brain and the nervous system, and outlines the main theories about why the body reacts as it does. Later chapters describe many of the common causes of pain, explain how pain is diagnosed and offer a brief insight into some of the orthodox and non-orthodox treatments available. It may feel like reading a medical textbook at times. However, the basic technical language and theoretical style in some sections are necessary to describe (as accurately and as simply as possible) *how* your body works. The better you are able to understand *why* you feel pain, the easier it may be to deal with the pain itself.

While this book cannot guarantee that you will become pain-free, it might help you discover how to manage your pain effectively. Draw from it whatever information and practical support you find useful. Look out for signposts to relevant sources of information and the addresses listed at the end of the book. A book carrying this type of information can be dipped in and out of wherever and whenever you choose; it doesn't have to be read strictly from cover to cover.

The information given in the case studies has been provided by people who genuinely suffer pain, many of whom are volunteer members of the national charity Action on Pain (see page 201). Other contributions have been made by relatives and colleagues of people with pain. The book has been directed primarily at you, the person with the pain, but it is inevitable that in many cases the wider family unit will also be affected. Some areas of the book acknowledge this – so if you feel that a relative may benefit from dipping into the book, then do share the information with them.

If your relative needs additional information, most of the organisations that deal with various illnesses also offer services that help to support relatives (see pages 201-210).

What have we learned over the centuries?

A brief history of pain would show that our sources of information have their origins in medical and social documentation, and in folklore. Early writers and thinkers believed that pain stemmed from our emotions, perhaps the result of an evil eye being cast upon us or punishment for a sin; others have suggested that it occurred because of an imbalance in body fluids or that feelings of pain emanated from the heart. Although we now know differently as far as physical pain is concerned, it is interesting that certain literary and colloquial expressions continue to focus on the heart as the organ responsible for unpleasant (painful) emotions. Think about such terms as 'heartfelt misery' and heroines suffering from a 'broken heart'.

Beliefs about how pain affects the body have developed gradually over the centuries; for example, an explanation given by the seventeenth century writer, Descartes, described a basic model of pain which linked the physical sensation felt on the skin to the brain as, 'a spark from a fire that stimulated threads in the skin to operate bells in the brain'. Modern scientists show that the route to the brain is less direct than Descartes' threads theory, although his reasoning was moving along the right lines, away from the heart-centred notion towards a nerve/brain connection.

In more recent times, the Gate Control Theory, published by Professors Melzack and Wall in 1965, drew together much information about how the body works, covering anatomical, biological, physiological and psychological functions of pain. Their views have helped to shed light on some of the complexity surrounding human perception of pain. Gate Control Theory, outlined on page 15, went a long way towards explaining the links between our sensory, our cognitive and our emotional processes. The theory has been updated (in 1982 and 1994) and is still recognised as a valid description of pain/nerve activity. It was noted earlier that each person responds differently by having an unalterable blueprint. We know that pain experienced even before we are born can imprint on our neurological system and shape the way we feel pain subsequently.

The experience and bearing of pain has long been seen as an inescapable part of being alive. Its very inevitability means that, by enduring pain, a human being could learn valuable lessons in mind and character development. Hence the advice, 'keep a stiff upper lip' and 'don't buckle under the strain', generally associated with maintaining self-control while suffering discomfort.

The saying 'no pain, no gain' is used regularly, particularly amongst sportsmen and women many of whom believe they must push their bodies beyond the 'pain barrier' before they can achieve their best athletic results. In some cultures this sentiment can also be found in tribal rituals where pain is inflicted but is seen as a 'rite of passage'; for example, the insertion of needles, jewellery or lying on a bed of nails. In all cultures, a powerful experience of extreme pain for many women is the pain of childbirth – an activity essential for the bringing forth of new life and ultimately the survival of the human species.

Whatever the origins and theories covering pain transmission, mankind has long sought to find remedies. Archaeological findings show that ancient medical practitioners first used poppy juice six centuries ago, in Sumerian times, as an antidote to pain. And extracts, derived from the opium poppy, albeit in more sophisticated forms, continue to be the key ingredient of strong painkilling drugs today. While plant-based remedies formed the mainstay of pain cures in Western societies, Oriental countries also developed therapies using touch, sensation and the practice of 'mind over matter', alongside their herbal remedies. Think, for example, about acupuncture, massage, hypnosis, Indian-style yoga and Ayurvedic remedies and how some of these methods are used to soothe and bring relief. Although there is less scientific evidence for the efficacy of many of these products and treatments (as found in Western-type studies), the treatments are practised extremely widely throughout the world. It is possible that the relief derived from non-plant therapies can at least be likened to (if not explained by) some aspects of Gate Control Theory. Complementary therapies are covered in greater detail in Chapter 5.

Consciousness and perception of pain

Our 'consciousness' has been described (by Hofstadter and Dennett in their book *The Mind's I)* as the 'most obvious and the most mysterious feature of our minds'. It is probably the place where we deliberate experiences, ponder ideas, enjoy sensations, formulate theories and 'view' perceptions – including suffering pain. It is believed that pain is an essential component of conscious existence, that all our sensations, thoughts and emotions are, in some form, associated with feelings of either pleasure or pain. In the former instance we try to replicate the sensation and in the latter we instinctively try to avoid repetition. Putting aside the perverse reasons why some people do otherwise, we view shunning pain as normal human behaviour. The desire to repeat pleasure needs no explanation and it is likely that the prime reason for avoiding pain is that of self-preservation, long embedded in our genetic make-up. An early caveman who survived a fight with a savage animal or stepped too close to the fire will have learned an abiding lesson.

In a physical and medical sense, people are considered to be either conscious or unconscious. Conscious people are (largely) in control of their feelings and actions, whereas an unconscious person (as far as we know) is not. It is probable that we need to be conscious to register sensations and perceptions of pain. However, these are conceptual ideas for which there is no empirical (true experiential) observation. What we do know is that perception of pain is a powerful physical and emotional entity, an integral and real part of our being. A glance at a dictionary shows a wide variety of words used commonly to describe pain and its effects upon our lives (see **Box 1**), and a quote from Oscar Wilde (*De Profundis*), made during the nineteenth century, suggests that pain is something that cannot easily be disguised:

> *'Behind joy and laughter there may be a temperament, coarse, hard and callous. But behind sorrow there is always sorrow. Pain, unlike pleasure, wears no mask.'*

Box 1 Describing pain

Words associated with pain include:		
Ache	Affliction	Agony
Anguish	Discomfort	Distress
Misery	Pang	Paroxysm
Suffering	Throes (of)	Torment
Torture	Twinge	Wretchedness
… and many more.		

What is pain and why do we feel it?

So how best can this imprecise thing called 'pain' be described and how does it manifest itself? Box 1 lists many words commonly associated with pain, illustrating how we might feel or how it might happen to affect us – but few words tell us what it actually is. The *Oxford English Dictionary* defines pain as, 'Bodily or mental suffering' and goes on to suggest that the word can be used to convey a number of meanings. These include 'penalty or punishment' as in 'pain of death', 'exertion' as in 'take pains to …', and several others.

Rather than defining pain as a concept and attempting to explain what it is, most medical textbooks, instead, tell us what it results from. In principle, medical opinion says that pain arises following:

- injury, due to accidental trauma;

- inflammation, stemming from an infection or similar pressure source in a body organ;

- surgery or a similar activity, which is medically induced.

These prime reasons for pain can then be categorised into many subdivisions and types, covered more fully in later chapters.

The role of pain is different to that of pressure caused by touch. All bodies (human and animal) have mechanisms that normally respond swiftly to the first trace of pain and various systems are programmed to recognise, react to, report on and try to remedy the feeling. At the first hint of a potential problem, triggered by the lightest of touches, a series of messages is despatched to the brain to ascertain whether the pressure felt by the skin is that of pain or pleasure. The overriding rationale is defensive, designed to avoid damage before real harm is done. The following examples broadly define 'threat avoidance':

- maintaining self-protection, such as preventing injury;

- alerting the body to developing disease, such as an infection in a wound;

- restricting the use of a body part, maybe because a bone is broken or a joint is inflamed as in arthritis;

- warning that a body part is malfunctioning, for example, when fluid builds up in the eye because the drainage exit is blocked (glaucoma);

- signalling the need to rest or slow down, perhaps indicated by a headache or, more seriously, an angina attack;

- warning that certain foods might be allergic or poisonous to our systems, for example, by causing a severe pain in the gut or, for some people, by setting off a migraine;

- stimulating avoidance action, for example, by blinking our eyes when we feel pain from looking directly at the sun.

Note: Many situations where pain is present call for immediate first aid and emergency action.

Gate Control Theory – how our body reacts

In basic, non-technical language, when body tissue is damaged pain impulses travel along special nerve fibres (explained more fully below) triggering the opening of a 'gateway'. The impulse carries the 'hurt' message first to a section of the spinal cord, called the dorsal horn, where the pain sensation pauses to interact with other nerves, before moving across the cord.

In most cases following an injury, the wounded individual (or another person) quickly takes action to relieve the pain. For example, if you knock your elbow you usually rub the affected area immediately. This soothing remedy is also transmitted to the dorsal horn area, along a different nerve pathway. Both types of nerve impulses then travel at great speed towards the brain, along *separate* routes, and the second set of sensations (the comforting feeling and warmth created by the rubbing action) actually travels faster, along a more direct route than the 'first' pain message along its designated pathway. The soothing sensation normally reaches the brain earlier than the discomfort alarm. Here, other controlling factors then play a part in influencing our perception about how severe the pain is.

Depending on the power of these influential sways, a 'gateway' is either shut or left open. When the former option is selected the painful sensation subsides; in the latter case it continues. It is believed that the pain gateway remains open under the influence of emotional inputs such as anxiety, excitement and fear, while cognitive inputs, such as distraction, calming words and imagery (for example, a mother's comforting behaviour or a self-generated message that says 'I'm OK') act to close the gate.

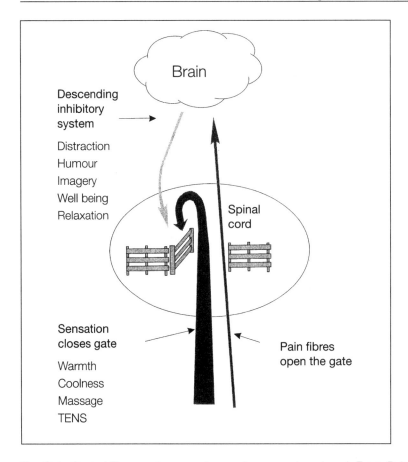

The Gate Control Theory – how a gate may be opened or closed. From *Pain: Creative approaches to effective management,* by Eloise Carr and Eileen Mann, published by Palgrave in 2000. Reproduced by kind permission of the authors and publisher.

If the discomfort is not relieved, the slower-moving pain signal is able to pass through the gateway to the brain. Gate Control Theory also helps to explain some of the more complex inconsistencies associated with pain perception, so it will be referred to again in later sections.

Sinead is a physiotherapist
'A simple way to practise Gate Control Theory is by remembering that touch overrides pain.'

The role of the brain and nervous system

The most important type of pain recognition is that caused by damage to the skin surface; for example, through a prick or compression or a burn. The sense governing pain is quite distinct from that of touch. Research has shown that all 'senses' picked up by the skin run up special nerve fibres in the spinal cord – those for pain travel near the central canal, whereas those for touch move through pathways in the posterior part of the cord. It is known that patients with the disease syringomyelia (a disorder affecting the central part of the spinal cord, see page 78) lose their sense of *pain* in their limbs, including heat and cold, but the slightest *touch* sense can still be felt.

The nerve endings for touch and pain, heat and cold are scattered thickly across the skin surface. It is probable that the receptors for these sensations are clustered in spots, as pain is felt with varying intensity at different places. All skin sensations that we describe are in fact variations of these basic senses. For example, an itch or a tickle is a form of touching, which can be produced by stimulating the skin with varying amounts of pressure or speed of movement. Any damage to body tissue triggers the production and release of chemicals, which react with each other and stimulate the nerve endings. The pain impulse then travels along designated routes via nerve fibres and is interpreted by the brain, as shown by the research discussed in Gate Control Theory (pages 15–16).

The (physical) action of nerves

There are three types of nerve fibres grouped according to three physiological rules: the type of message they transport, their size and their speed of activity. Two of the types (known as the A-delta and C fibres) carry pain sensations and the third type (called A-beta fibres) carry non-pain messages, derived from warmth and touch.

The A-delta fibres are responsible for the swift reactions (reflex responses) that occur when we are exposed to immediate harm, such as burning skin. This acute pain is called 'first' or 'fast' pain and travels very quickly to the brain via the dorsal horn of the spinal cord. The message is received in the specific brain cortex area where it is immediately interpreted and the source located. It is this 'interpretation' or 'perception' which gives rise to the complexity of pain as it involves an emotional and cognitive element as well as the physical. In other words, it is affected by a dual situation (ie how we are feeling and the *meaning* of the pain). The experience of pain is multidimensional and the value of the Gate Control Theory is that it allows us to see pain with these different components in mind. These A-delta fibres also recognise the merest pinprick-like sensations and this mechanism remains present, even after general pain senses have been dulled by strong drugs. This sense remains because there are no 'opioid' receptors on their surface. (Opioid receptors are points at which opium-like substances, whether produced internally by the body or given as a drug, can become attached.) This pain-sensitive action acts as another defensive mechanism to help protect the body, and its highly attuned sense can be over-ridden only by nerve-blocking procedures or an anaesthetic.

The C fibres conduct pain more slowly than A-delta fibres and are responsible for the type of pain known as 'second' pain. It usually follows the sharp pain and feels like a gnawing, throbbing sensation, which spreads over a wider location. The C fibres share the same nerve pathways as the A-delta fibres but end up being interpreted in a more generalised area of the brain, at its stem. C fibre-type pain is responsive to strong, opioid (opium-like) drugs.

The A-beta fibres, also found on the surface of the skin, are the largest and swiftest acting of the three types and are triggered by non-painful touch and sensation. Their fast passage to the brain is significant to the reasoning behind Gate Control Theory. A-beta fibres get to the brain more quickly than either the A-delta fibres or C fibres because they enter the dorsal horn area of the spinal cord on the same side as they leave it, thus travelling by a more direct and faster route. Although A-delta and C fibres enter at the same point, they must first pass across the dorsal horn to leave from the opposite side. It might seem odd that 'soothing' senses get to the brain more speedily than messages indicating pain, but that is how it appears to be. It certainly seems to stop our bodies from over-reacting to every little sensation.

It seems also that, although the responses to (and feelings generated by) pain are normally different, several research studies have shown that, if pain remains untreated, the nerves can 'cross wires' and send signals that do not correspond to the original stimulus, so that a soft touch actually feels painful. Think back to when you last had a very bad bout of pain that was not treated adequately. You may remember your whole body beginning to feel sore, even to the touch of clothing.

The (physical) action of pain chemicals

Any painful skin incident produces a chemical reaction instantly in the bloodstream, generating a series of substances that immediately come into contact with the nerve receptors just below the skin surface. Some of these chemicals help to trigger feelings of instantaneous pain, but once the process has been initiated, the site of the injury goes on being perceptive to pain by continuing to produce more chemicals. These additional chemicals strengthen the pain conduction to the brain, thus increasing sensitivity. This phenomenon helps to explain why an injured area remains sore for days after the trauma. The term 'hyperalgesia' is used to describe extreme sensitivity to pain. A different term, 'allodynia', is applied when the stimulus, such as light clothing, would not normally provoke pain (see the section on shingles, page 75).

Conversely, and here is another example of the complexity of the pain process and the magic of the body's resources, a separate chemical action is taking place at the same time to reduce or remove the effects of pain. This pain reduction process is known as 'pain modulation'. Firstly, the function of some substances appears to inhibit the action of enzymes called 'prostaglandins', which play an important role in the production of pain. (You may hear about prostaglandins elsewhere as they play many other roles in the body.) A second element of pain modulation is the production of opioid-type chemicals in the body. These internally-produced, opium-like chemicals are called 'endogenous' opioids and they work particularly to suppress nerve impulses and dampen down the perception of pain in the different brain centres. The action of many analgesic (pain-reducing) drugs mimics those produced naturally by the body and much pharmaceutical research is based on pain modulation theory.

Clare is a GP
'When the body is trying to repair itself simultaneously in several different places, the healing process naturally takes longer because the resources have to be spread around.'

The diversity of pain

Internal organs and the deeper layers of skin are much less sensitive to pain than the surface and upper layers. Internal organs have more protection and any discomfort felt here tends to be perceived differently, as these areas do not possess the ability to feel the type of pain caused by sudden injury. It may be difficult to believe but once the skin surface had been severed it would be possible to cut through a section of bowel without a person knowing, provided their view was obstructed. Tendon, muscle and bone are also less sensitive to pain under normal circumstances; however, inflammatory reaction in these parts and changes to their function can influence interpretation by the brain, causing immense distress. Hence the severe pain felt when a limb is broken.

When an injury or build up of inflammation or a blockage occurs in any internal (and dense) structure found inside the body, the pain felt is actually due to congestion caused by swollen blood vessels or fluid or pus pressing on surrounding nerves and other organs. The pain felt in these circumstances is much more likely to be described as a throbbing sensation, rather than the sharp flash of pain from injury to the skin.

Where the space is very confined, such as ears or eyes, the pain is very intense and localised. Patients with pain in their bones use words such as gnawing, and pain caused by a tumour pressing on or invading surrounding tissue might be spoken of as boring or piercing. Over-use of muscles or over-stretching of a weaker body part causes a tender ache, such as that felt in calf muscles after an arduous walk, or the tight spasm, often called a 'stitch', which appears at the side of the abdomen after strenuous exercise. Both these types of pain are due partly to deposits of irritating chemicals, which build up after intense bouts of activity.

Nerve pain (neuralgia) gives severe and constant discomfort. Irritation of the bowel, as in irritable bowel syndrome or colic, is griping in nature, similar to pain in the ureters and bile ducts; while a blockage in any of these organs, caused by an impassable object such as a kidney or gall stone or bulky stool causes agonising pain due to the compression of nerves and surrounding tissue. Burning pain can be caused by the acidic action of gastric fluids found in various types of abdominal ulcers or regurgitation of stomach contents in hiatus hernia or dyspepsia (indigestion). Any condition can become painful if an organ is subjected to excess damage; for example, the effects of strong light or loud noise produce painful sensations.

Emily's story

Emily has arthritis and describes it partly as a 'deterioration of parts with age'. She says that although it could be called 'pain' it is more like a severe discomfort, allied to stiffness. The problems have been present for twenty years but increasingly so in the last ten years.

On poor days Emily has mostly lower back and neck pain, with pain also in her arms, legs, hands and feet now and then. She says it is most uncomfortable after she starts to move when she has been immobile for a while, perhaps sitting for extensive periods in a chair or lying in bed. She also finds that standing still for a long time or after a lengthy walk increases the discomfort in her back. Fortunately, general movements and varied activities such as housework or gardening are all right while she is doing the job – the discomfort tends to appear afterwards when she is sitting down. It feels like a generalised pain, rather than sharp specific pangs, and slows her down.

Mostly exercise helps, and Emily is able to cycle quite a bit. As a real bonus, she also enjoys Scottish dancing once a week. She admits that she grumbles a bit about her difficulties.

For Emily, the three key words that spring to mind in relation to her illness are 'nagging', 'depressing' and 'nuisance'.

Like the majority of pain sufferers, Emily believes that her discomfort affects those around her, mainly because it limits their choice of what to do. She says, rather succinctly, 'short walk – yes; long walk – no'.

The treatment(s) that have worked best for Emily over the years have been a combination of medication and therapies from the following lists:

Prescribed by the general practitioner or hospital consultant

- *Various anti-inflammatory drugs (at present diclofenac sodium 75mg) – used for rheumatoid and musculo-skeletal disorder and gout. Emily says she does not like to take drugs constantly.*
- *Exercises – as advised by the 'back school' at the hospital – to help get in and out of bed and for her back, neck, knees, ankles and toes.*

Self-help treatments
- *Swimming (which was also suggested by her doctor)*
- *Cod liver oil.*

Complementary therapies
- *None tried.*

Emily has never been referred to a pain clinic. She feels that it would be nice to be more informed about causes and remedies (if any exist) or anything that would help her arthritis. She believes that 'better understanding' usually helps.

Behavioural responses to pain

Pain makes people react differently and their behaviour or emotional response is likely to relate to a combination of factors, depending on the nature and cause of the pain, how long it has been present and how severe it is. But, despite individual levels of response, human behaviour and experience resulting from pain generally tends to follow similar lines. Think about what reactions or outcomes have resulted from your own pain, or the pain of someone close to you. Box 2 lists a few examples, there are many more.

Box 2 Outcomes of pain

Pain is often blamed for (or produces) many of the following outcomes:		
Alcohol and drug misuse	Anger	Break-up of a relationship
Clumsiness	Discomfort	Exhaustion
Fear	Irritability	Isolation
Lost job or early retirement	Nausea	Self-harm and suicide
Untruthfulness	Violence	Withdrawal
Note: Pain assessment is covered more fully in Chapter 3.		

Julia and Martin

Martin and his wife Julia are both in their early 60s, and have been happily married for over 35 years. Three years ago, Julia developed trigeminal neuralgia which caused her intense pain in the face. Martin was shocked by the change in his bright, capable wife.

'Of course it was horrible seeing her so ill,' he confided in a friend. 'But the worst thing was what the pain did to her. Suddenly, she had aged dramatically – she seemed about a hundred! She's always been so strong and organised. I didn't know what to do ...'

Fortunately, Julia's condition cleared up spontaneously, and only then did Martin feel able to admit just how scared he had been. 'I suppose my greatest fear was not that she'd die, but that she just wouldn't get better. I couldn't recognise the woman I'd been married to for all these years.'

Psychological (emotional and cognitive) aspects of pain

Psychology (the study of the mind) now touches almost every facet of our lives. As society has become more complex, so the science of psychology has assumed a greater role in explaining the meaning of human behaviour and in solving some of its problems. Psychologists can show that pain will activate behaviours that override most other stimuli. Avoidance of pain, the survival mechanism whereby living creatures react to stay away from danger, can also be linked to an inherent compulsion to continue the existence of that species as a living organism.

There are lots of different ways in which the so-called 'psychological' aspects of pain can be described, so a few examples will be covered here as illustrations only. We are aware that pain manifests itself in two ways, as both physical and psychological elements, which are interlinked. The original trauma sets off a biological process, which ends in the discernible feeling we call pain. Scientists know quite a lot about the physical experience because it is now relatively easy to study physiological processes. The psychological element is less easy to explain because it takes place in our minds and, as yet, researchers are unable to view how the mind works in the same tangible way. However, some form of mental activity is evidently taking place. The connection between the two systems was described earlier in Gate Control Theory. Scientists are confident that mental and emotional influences, such as fear and anxiety, depression, past experiences, our ability to take control of the situation, are very significant and play a major part in controlling our perception about the severity of pain.

The cognitive element – our interpretation and understanding – takes place in the higher centres of the brain and is an important area, one where many people will feel empathy. Essentially, the cognitive element is what gives pain its *meaning*. Therapies such as 'cognitive behaviour therapy' (CBT – see page 130) are used to address the fears associated with particular types of pain, and help us to develop coping strategies. Back pain is a good example as it can be very alarming. People are often fearful of activity, believing it might damage their spine and make the situation worse. Therefore they reduce their activity. However, we now know that this approach is generally unhelpful. Another example is that of chest pain – a young woman might shrug this off as indigestion, but a man whose father has died of a heart attack may instantly fear his chest pain indicates he too is having heart problems.

The mystery of pain

Pain can be triggered by illusory as well as real experiences. There are reported examples of people describing uncomfortable sensations and even overwhelming pain, without an obvious physical cause. If we perceive pain through conscious thought as described earlier perhaps it's possible that the brain plays 'tricks' – mental concepts with physical manifestations.

> *'A person may suffer pain without any external cause, the mind misinterpreting or exaggerating sensation ...'* (Black's Medical Dictionary)

This does not imply that, if a person feels pain for no identifiable reason, then the pain is not real. Nor does it mean that the person is mentally ill and experiencing delusions of pain. Patients who have had a limb amputated frequently describe the sensation of pain in an extremity that no longer exists. Perhaps even more strangely, the discomfort can be felt, not immediately after the trauma which might be expected, but many years later (see phantom pain, page 39).

Pain is recognised as a 'subjective' entity and it is therefore difficult to define it 'objectively'. Attempts have been made by several authors to characterise the feeling, favouring either the patients' or the medical viewpoint, for example:

Pain is …

> *'Whatever the experiencing person says it is and existing whenever he says it does.'*(McCaffery and Beebe, 1994)

or

> *'An unpleasant sensory and emotional experience associated with actual or potential tissue damage, or describing in terms of such damage.'* (International Association for the Study of Pain (IASP), 1986)

The IASP also points out that pain may exist without tissue damage.

In a different sense, people who talk about the emotional hurt they are feeling after an emotional shock, such as bereavement or an horrific experience, are also describing a form of psychologically induced pain. The anguish caused by this mental feeling, derived from sadness or terror, is just as real as that caused by a tangible wound, even though its presence flouts sensible assumptions because there is no damage to flesh or nerves. However, the triggering event is real and the body may equally show signs associated with physical trauma; for example, aching limbs, nausea, shaking and soreness.

The placebo effect

The 'placebo effect' is a phenomenon founded on a psychological premise. The word 'placebo' translated from the Latin means *I will please* and historically in medicine placebos were given to pacify patients even when there were no known, obvious benefits. A medical placebo is an inert compound that has no action. The inactive substances when taken did no harm and often achieved positive results because the patients assumed, through psychological belief, they were being treated by an effective cure. Doctors are well aware that the psychological perception of *feeling* better is often accompanied by positive physical signs that indicate the person is *getting* better; for example, positive changes can be recorded in blood pressure levels and pulse rates. Improved pain results have also been reported as a result of placebo treatments and a reduction in psychological symptoms, anxiety and insomnia in particular, are common.

This placebo response is seen often enough to make doctors respect its effect and is thought to be brought about by the reassurance factor – the conviction that actually taking something for the problem is bound to be advantageous. This therapeutic belief placed on the value of a treatment is still present in society today as, on the whole, we expect a drug or therapy to 'do us good'. It also remains a fact that like our forebears we are susceptible to persuasion and are still capable of being deceived – by our own thoughts, as well as by claims made by unscrupulous practitioners.

The placebo experience has a very important role in modern research. Placebos, in the form of chemically inert substances, are given to patients as an essential part of any drug testing experiment, to help establish the usefulness of the real drug being tested. A form of 'double-blind' research is usually performed. In the first part of the double-blind procedure one set of patients in the trial is randomly selected by computer and given the true drug and the other group is given an identical looking tablet with biologically neutral qualities. The second blind factor is that the nurses who administer the drugs do not know which patients are being given which version – this information is known only to the researchers. Similarly, studies into therapeutic, psychological treatments are also subjected to rigorous control procedures. Throughout both types of research, opportunities do exist for manipulation – which could leave the whole process open to misunderstanding and inaccurate conclusions. Whether it is a drug company testing new pills or people promoting a new form of therapy, it could be argued they have a vested interest in wishing their treatment to be successful.

Here lies the pertinent question – how do the people doing the research prove that the individuals taking part have been truly helped by the treatment and not influenced by the placebo effect? Because it does have the power to influence the results quite significantly, this effect cannot be ignored and strict testing must be established to eliminate poor practice. However, the placebo effect is well understood (and in itself well researched) so when the results are analysed the researchers know how to take into account accurately the psychological bias and to eliminate its effects. The researchers are required to demonstrate conclusively before a new product is accepted that the people taking part in the study had actually improved as a result of the drug or psychological treatment, and not because they had merely imagined they felt better.

Care is taken when placebos are used in trials dealing with acute pain – for two reasons. Firstly, some patients when given the placebo tablet do seem to obtain noticeable pain relief, not because of the placebo effect, but because their pain, present at the start of the trial, may have subsided naturally, so this effect must be accounted for. However, as we have seen already nothing about pain is simple; and other experiments have shown that some people who receive a placebo, and experience a reduction of their pain, actually get their pain back again when they are given a drug called naloxone which reverses the effect of opioids. What has been suggested is that some people are sensitive to the 'placebo effect'. This means that taking the placebo actually causes their bodies to produce their own endogenous opioids (endorphins) and it is these which are largely responsible for the reduction of their pain.

Secondly, some patients who are given the analgesic drug get no pain relief so it would be unethical to allow them to continue suffering. In all cases, if the pain does not settle, additional analgesics are given.

Product licences for drugs are awarded only after strict clinical trials have been carried out to check the effectiveness and safety of all medication. As part of this process, which can take years, all research studies are subjected to something called 'peer review'. The methods used are care-fully checked for any flaws by fellow medical experts and colleagues and in some cases, where there are doubts, they may repeat the research. Claims for authentic cures are not substantiated until responsible people are sure beyond reasonable doubt of their reliability. It would be false to say that results are right every time, because on rare occasions harmful treatments have slipped through the safety net. On balance, new drugs and therapies are very unlikely to enter into mainstream medicine before their safety is assured.

Maggie's story

Maggie has arthritis in both knees which has developed over the last ten years, since she 'slipped a disc'. Maggie says the pain is mostly constant, really a bad ache that is affected very much by the weather. Damp weather Maggie finds especially a nuisance as that 'brings the pain on' more severely.

As the arthritis has worsened, Maggie can no longer squat or sit cross-legged, something that she did regularly before. Going up stairs is relatively easy but going down stairs is something that she avoids at all costs, wherever possible. Having to step down from a high step also cause problems and running and jogging are now out of the question – although Maggie does find that walking helps.

The expressions Maggie uses to describe how she feels are 'irritated' and 'it stops me from doing such a lot of things'.

The treatments that have worked best for Maggie over the years have been a combination of self-help medication and activities.

Maggie says that she does not like taking any type of drugs so she has not asked for medical help from her doctor. Normally, she says, she puts up with the condition. However, about three months before writing this little piece about her arthritis, she came across an article in a health magazine mentioning the food supplement glucosamine. She bought a bottle of tablets and within six weeks felt the pain in her knees had reduced. She acknowledges that the improvement could have been because she had taken up swimming again and was walking more, but she believes that the main benefit has come from the glucosamine. Maggie has recently returned from Iraq where she stayed for three weeks. On the second day there she gave the bottle of tablets to an older lady to take as she was also in a lot of pain in her knees from arthritis. Because Maggie had not been taking the food supplement she felt the pain in her knees had got worse. The first thing Maggie did when she returned to England was to go along to the health food shop and buy herself another bottle of glucosamine.

Auto-suggestion

The good news is that in an everyday context the placebo benefit can still be used to good effect because positive psychological factors, such as hope, expectation of improvement and receiving attention, are very important components in the overall treatment process. Although spectacular achievements have been made in technical equipment and drug therapy, an important element remains the trust patients put into the words spoken by medical practitioners. This is not to suggest that people are being fooled by what a doctor says. It is more about one seeming to work better when supported by the other. Similarly, where faith healers attempt to restore health by direct mental suggestion, the fact that people are open to desiring a 'good' result plays a very significant role in the outcome. In another sense, a personal belief in the power of self-help is an important factor which is known to help the body heal itself.

The relief of pain through psychological methods has been attributed to the fact that the person may have been suffering (sometimes for many years) from a condition known as 'pithiatism', a form of hysteria where the symptoms are 'due to auto-suggestion and are readily relieved by suggestion from another person' *(Black's Medical Dictionary)*. To link pain to a condition such as hysteria might have uncomfortable implications for some, as hysteria in previous times was thought to be linked to women's problems (*hustera* was the Greek word for womb). The problems were thought to be due to an over-reaction of some parts of the nervous system, causing the body to mimic other organic disorders.

Whatever term is used, hysterical-type reactions did, and still do, occur. People are known to exhibit mentally-induced changes such as convulsive seizures, paralysis and loss of feeling, without obvious medical illness; muscle spasms and limb contractions are examples of hysteria-linked, non-organic disorders capable of causing severe discomfort. Much more is now known about psychiatric illness, where symptoms described by patients do not always have an identifiable cause.

Psycho-social (cultural) implications

The trauma of pain is rarely confined to individual suffering. Doctors are aware that the pain and suffering of a family member can have a huge impact on their loved ones. After visiting their GP or hospital consultant, the patient will be keen to report what the doctor said and equally, most family members will listen to their account and ask relevant questions, because reassurance about progress or assurance that the problem is not serious, are joyful news. Conversely, a bulletin that contains poor news inevitably impacts on those close by. Pain is an emotion that crosses personal boundaries and is capable of generating quite strong psycho-social consequences and we know that some forms of chronic pain result in considerable impact on the family unit. If a child is suffering, its parents also suffer. If one partner is in pain, the other partner is usually all too aware of their misery and feels miserable too.

Jane's story

Jane has endured spinal stenosis for 39 years. She says that she has good days and bad days but, although the good days are great, they are dangerous as it makes her feel that she should be doing more to make up for the days when she can't do anything. She then worries about her muscles weakening. Bad days far outnumber the good days and they can vary enormously, right down to not being able to get out of bed. Enough of these days in a row causes bad depression, feelings of worthlessness and of being a burden.

Jane says the pain is mostly in her spine, lumbar and cervical regions but very often it affects her shoulders, arms, hands and hips. It also causes severe migraine, which can last 4-5 days.

For Jane, the three key words that spring to mind in relation to her illness are 'depression', 'frustration' and 'helplessness'.

Jane says that the pain affects her family and friends by curtailing their social life and it means that planned events often have to be cancelled at the last minute.

The treatment(s) that have worked best for Jane over the years have been a combination of medication and therapies from the following lists:

Prescribed by the general practitioner or hospital consultant	Self-help treatments	Complementary therapies
Non-steroidal anti-inflammatory drugs (NSAIDs) and painkillers	*Pacing herself*	*Aromatherapy*
Acupuncture	*Swimming*	*Self-hypnosis*
Hydrotherapy	*Yoga*	*Massage*
Botox		
Supra-scapula nerve block injections		
Facet joint injections		
Traction		

Jane feels that attending a pain clinic definitely helped. She thinks that the most valuable thing that she learned was 'pacing'. Before learning to do this she had felt that not finishing a task was admitting defeat.

FACT BOX

- About 10 per cent of people in Western countries report suffering from chronic pain *(Bandolier's Little Book of Pain)*.

- More than 6,000 patients are treated annually at the NHS Centre for Pain Relief at Walton in Liverpool, Europe's biggest pain-relieving clinic (Pain Research Institute).

- Pain can become 'chronic' in as little as four weeks (see page 37) but is more generally accepted as being chronic after three months.

- About 45-50 per cent of patients attending GP run (community-based) pain clinics report symptoms of low back pain and sciatica *(Pain Bulletin,* Pain Research Institute).

- Arthritis pain increases dramatically with age to afflict a quarter of people aged 60 or over *(Bandolier's Little Book of Pain)*.

- If even 10 per cent of the population had pain every day (likely from a Scottish survey by Elliott in 1999) then there would be over 2 billion days of pain per year in the UK. That is 30-40 days of pain for every one of us *(Bandoliers Little Book of Pain)*.

Conclusion

People often assume that they must 'live with their pain', which begs the question 'must this be so'? The answer, of course, is not clear cut. Yes, pain will always be a factor in human make-up, a very essential part of our being because it has a meaning, warning us that something is wrong, but…it is unacceptable that people suffer. The World Health Organization, which sees the pain and suffering world wide, believes that relief from pain is a basic human right. However, many people in the UK continue to suffer needlessly due to a multitude of factors.

As this chapter has shown, pain is a complex issue – felt largely in a physical sense but controlled and influenced by centres in the brain which scientists still know little about. Without an ability to feel pain, our defences would be severely compromised. Mild to moderate pain, while unpleasant in the first instance, can be easily remedied with an armoury of pills and ointments, many of which are available over the counter, without the need to consult a doctor. Non-steroidal anti-inflammatory drugs (NSAIDs, see Chapter Four) can give such effective pain relief they are second only to some of the opioids. Many people seek interventions for the relief of their pain, or to help them cope better with their pain, from practitioners outside of the medical arena.

More severe pain, and that caused by chronic disease or a deteriorating body function, is more wearing and more likely to need medical attention. It is worth noting that we are likely to see an increase in the prevalence of chronic pain as it is associated with many disease processes, such as arthritis, which are more likely to manifest as we grow older. The good news is that there are now a wealth of interventions, from analgesics to relaxation strategies, that can be used to help us manage pain more effectively. Ingenious mankind has come up with many physical and psychological solutions to lessen the force and learning how to live with pain is a much less formidable journey than in former times. Good pain control is achievable.

The following chapter looks at different types of pain, pain caused by cancer and the common causes of non-malignant pain.

For more information

Internet websites
For readers who have access to the Internet, a huge number of websites are available dealing with pain, offering users a range of information and facilities, covering evidence-based research, editorial comment, chat rooms, book reviews and self-help advice. Many are international, not all offer a permanent service and readers should be aware that there is no regulatory body protecting Internet users. The following examples are British-based sites that readers might wish to investigate. See also the address list starting on page 201:

* **NHS Direct Online**: www.nhsdirect.nhs.uk
  Provides quality information and advice on a wide range of health issues and disorders.

- **National Electronic Library of Health (NeLH)** www.nelh.nhs.uk
  Some information on this site is limited to health professionals only.

- **Cochrane Library**: www.update.software.com
  The Cochrane Library is an electronic publication designed to supply high quality evidence to people providing and receiving care. It is published quarterly on CD-ROM and the Internet after payment of a subscription fee.

- **Bandolier**: www.bandolier.com
  Provides evidenced-based health care advice and information.

- **Oxford Pain Internet Site**: www.jr2.ox.ac.uk/bandolier
  This site is connected to the Oxford Pain Relief Unit (the home of Bandolier and Pain Research) based at the Churchill Hospital, Oxford. Part of the NHS, the Unit treats patients from central England, elsewhere in the UK and from abroad.

- **Action on Pain**: www.action-on-pain.co.uk (see page 201)

- **The Pain Relief Foundation**: www.painrelieffoundation.org.uk (see also below)

- **The British Pain Society**: www.britishpainsociety.org (see page 203)

- **Pain Support UK**: www.painsupport.co.uk (see page 208).

Books and leaflets

- *Bandolier's Little Book of Pain,* Oxford University Press. This book is aimed at professional workers, providing an evidence-based guide to treatments; it would be useful for readers who wish to take an academic approach to studying pain.

- *Escape from Pain,* by Oliver Gillie (1997). Self-Help Direct Publishing.

- HELPBOX (The Help for Health Trust): provides a computer database of health-related information (see address on page 205).

- The Pain Relief Foundation (see address on page 208) is a charity that focuses on fighting pain through research, education and information. It runs a Pain Research Institute and offers a wide range of leaflets and a *Pain Bulletin* newsletter.

- *The Science of Suffering,* by Patrick Wall (1999). Weidenfeld & Nicolson.

2 Pain – types and common causes

Chapter One introduced you to some of the reasons why pain occurs and how it might affect your body. This chapter will continue explaining some of the multi-dimensional characteristics by describing types of pain. The latter part of the chapter takes a look at some of the more common causes of pain. It should perhaps be pointed out at this stage that, because this is a general book, the particular disorder that causes your pain may not be covered very fully – indeed it may not actually be mentioned at all.

But this does not make it any the less important.

As we have seen in Chapter One, the topic of 'pain' is very complex and the key information applies to all causes. The text should go a long way towards answering your questions and it may also raise uncertainties about other issues. Later chapters will define 'levels' or severity of pain, look more precisely at how it is assessed and point you towards other sources of help where you may find answers.

Types of pain

A basic understanding of pain categories will be a useful tool when you need to consult with a professional person. Whatever their status – a medical doctor, the practice nurse at your surgery or health centre, or a practitioner in complementary therapies, such as an aromatherapist or chiropractor – they will all use a similar language to illustrate pain. Adopting a common terminology helps enormously when you are discussing problems and treatments. But if you are unsure what a word means don't try to guess, ask for an explanation, no one will mind. The IASP (International Association for the Study of Pain) offers clear classification but, for simplicity, the following basic descriptions have been used. The order has no bearing on importance or severity. There is a misguided belief that acute pain is seen as more important than chronic (which is not true) or that chronic pain can't be acute, which it can.

Acute pain

Acute pain in this context means 'sharp' or 'penetrating' or 'keen'. In mathematics, an acute angle is one that is narrow and pointed; it comes from the Latin word *acus,* meaning needle. Acute pain has a number of recognisable characteristics, which help doctors make a diagnosis. Acute pain is:

- related to some sort of trauma or swiftly developing disease (for example, a broken limb or appendicitis);

- sudden in onset (over a few hours) with the most severe pain felt during the initial 24 hours;

- relatively short in timespan (maybe 2-3 days unless the problem is treated or it heals naturally but swiftly); if the problem is not treated either a crisis occurs (such as a burst appendix) or the severe pain gradually subsides to moderate pain over about five days (as the body starts to heal); it rarely lasts longer than two or three weeks.

Acute pain would be found in many situations where a severe infection or inflammation is building up. These may include an abscess or cholecystitis (inflammation of the gall bladder, see page 59), or where a blockage is causing pressure on surrounding tissues, for example, the movement of a kidney stone (see page 73), or where a wound has been caused either by accidental injury or through intended surgery. The inflammation tends to be localised and is a protective measure in response to the injury or to the presence of foreign material, such as the increased levels of bacteria (and pus) found at the site of an infection.

The purpose of the inflammation is to separate the injury (or diseased area) from whatever is causing the problem. The body does this in a number of ways: by forming a barrier with new tissue (part of the clotting process), or by destroying the harmful material with antibodies, or by diluting the poison with fluid. These attacking measures lead to four main signs and symptoms:

- **Pain** from pressure.

- **Redness** from increased blood brought to the area.

- **Heat** to kill the bacteria.

- **Swelling** from increased fluid.

These indicators will usually improve swiftly when some form of intervention halts the spread, either through natural healing or medically based treatments (see below). Even an abscess feels better after it has burst because the pressure is reduced. A word of caution however: waiting for the natural process to take its course is rarely a wise option. Any situation involving a suspected infection should always be investigated. An untreated infection can quickly develop into a very serious and sometimes fatal illness, as happened all too often before the discovery of antibiotics.

Chronic pain

The term 'chronic' pain relates to its longer-lasting nature because the pain remains present (albeit in a different form) after the original, acute injury or illness has cleared up. The defining, medical characteristics depict a type of pain that:

- lasts usually for more than a month (however, timing definitions do vary so the pain may have become 'chronic' at an earlier stage – see below);

- may be constant or sporadic, but probably present more often than it is absent;

- may not have an identifiable cause.

Chronic pain is likely to be found in situations where curative treatments are less easy to perform; for example, where the nerve associated with the pain is lying adjacent to a vital organ, such as sciatic pain, coming from the sciatic nerve which runs close to the spinal cord (see page 75). The signs and symptoms found in chronic pain will vary depending on their cause; different disorders give different kinds of indicators and intensities, many of which will be covered later in this chapter.

For more precise identification and a guide to treatment, chronic pain is further sub-divided into two categories:

- chronic *non*-malignant pain, such as arthritis, is continuing and has no foreseeable cut off point;

- chronic malignant pain can be ended, for example by appropriate treatment.

The minimum time span before discomfort is characterised varies, as specialists in the field define chronic pain differently. In a Scottish-based study it was described as 'pain or discomfort that persisted continuously or intermittently for longer than three months' *(Bandolier's Little Book of Pain)*. In this study about 5,000 questionnaires were distributed to people in a community setting, with four fifths of people returning their forms. Half of the respondents said they had chronic pain, with severity that increased with age. The most common reasons given were arthritis (see pages 46–50), back pain (see page 51) and angina (see page 44). IASP (International Association for the Study of Pain) in its *Classification of Chronic Pain* (1986), used the three-month time frame also.

Opinions differ and more recent observations (including a study by Weddell in 1992) suggested that acute back pain could become chronic within days due to muscle wastage and loss of bone density. A later study (carried out by Potter in 1998) found that three months was also too long and reduced the suggested time period to less than four weeks. Certainly, prolonged pain can develop from problems initially caused by acute pain, eg where a bone heals awkwardly following a complicated fracture, or where damaged tendons continue to ache after a sports injury.

John had multiple fractures after an accident
'The pain was constant for weeks, despite regular doses of painkillers. The morphine never quite suppressed the background pain.'

Cancer pain

This pain is caused by a developing malignant tumour as found in a cancerous growth. The topic is covered more fully on pages 41–43.

The nature of pain

The following descriptions are commonly used to differentiate between different patterns of pain.

Intermittent pain

As the name implies, this is pain that occurs erratically and often at infrequent intervals.

Intractable pain

This is pain that is difficult to manage, ease or control, in an effective way.

Persistent pain

This is pain that continues without letting up, in a steady and unrelenting manner.

Phantom pain

This is the name given to the pain that appears to be coming from a body part no longer present, for example following limb amputation, mastectomy and hernia. The true reasons are not fully understood but research suggests that it originates from the peripheral section of the severed nerve and continues to be felt because of changes within the brain or spinal cord (see also pages 24–25). Some of the antidepressant drugs are very helpful for neuropathic pain such as this, but again their precise way of working is not fully understood.

Referred pain

This type of pain is relatively common and can be confusing. When pain originates from the skin surface, the nerves and brain work in conjunction to pinpoint quite accurately the source of the problem (because pain is felt naturally and easily from the skin). However, if the source of the pain is an internal organ, unaccustomed to registering unpleasant sensations, the central nervous system plays further tricks. The mind transfers the feeling to a point where pain is more usually felt, because the nerve fibres share the same routes. For example, early pain coming from a damaged hip joint may be felt around the inner thigh and knee areas; and pain from internal organs may appear to be felt in quite remote and unlikely spots. Where referred pain might be expected during the course of an illness, its manner and usual site will be noted under the appropriate condition, later in the chapter.

Secondary pain

This is felt more as a dull ache which radiates across an area usually after the first, sharp pain has subsided. It might occur after an inflamed, localised spot, the main site of an infection, has been prodded.

Somatic pain

This describes pain originating in the musculo-skeletal system, relating to muscles, bones, joints, tendons and ligaments, although the word actually means 'relating to the body'. Its opposite would be 'psychosomatic' pain, a term sometimes used in connection with imagined pain depicted during episodes of mental stress.

Tractable pain

This is pain that is easily controlled.

Visceral pain

This is pain originating from internal organs found in the thoracic, abdominal and pelvic cavities.

Treatments

Today, pain is most likely to be improved by treatment, usually through medical intervention, but also as self-administered remedies. Obvious examples include: taking a course of antibiotics, using painkilling drugs (either prescribed by a doctor or bought over-the-counter), corrective surgery, immobilising the damaged part of the body and, conversely, by exercising to improve muscle and joint movement and strength, and using complementary therapies and self-help treatments. Treatments differ according to several factors – the reason for the pain, the type of pain present, the urgency of the situation – and they are usually given in combination. There are several significant factors that influence how doctors might proceed with various treatment options. One of these is whether or not the pain is being caused by a cancerous (malignant) growth or a benign (non-malignant) growth; a second factor is where in the body the pain is coming from, because investigating or operating in some areas carries a much higher risk than in other areas that are easily accessible.

Typical treatments for each disorder are given briefly under its heading in the section below and treatments in general are covered more fully in Chapters Four and Five.

Pain caused by cancer

So much is now known about cancer that the topic demands whole books to itself, and they are readily available in bookshops for people who need this type of specialist knowledge and advice. However, in a book about pain, this illness does require particular mention, and specific detail will be included where appropriate. The section below refers only to cancer, describing what it is and how it develops. The explanation is technical in parts, so if it is not of any interest to you then feel free to jump straight to the next part of the book (page 43). By doing so, you will not miss any other important information.

Cancer is not a single disease as the name suggests, but a general term covering over two hundred different types of malignant tumours sharing common factors. Each type of cancer is distinctive, with its own symptoms and characteristics determined by the sort of tumour involved, and where it arises in the body. All cancers start in the same way when the information that controls the growth of a normal body cell goes wrong. The message to the cell is altered and, from this point onwards, that cell grows abnormally. In fact this abnormal process happens regularly but the body usually recognises very early on that something is wrong and destroys the rogue cell. When a cancer develops, it is because the body has failed to detect the problem and gradually the flawed cells divide and increase until a cluster or lump of cells builds up. Cells are very small in size so it takes a lot of abnormal cell division before a collection of unusual cells gives noticeable symptoms and the presence of a growth (tumour) is diagnosed.

Because the body is constructed from cells, technically a cancer could develop in every living part. In reality malignant tumours tend to grow more readily in certain areas and that is because more than one element is necessary. The following list includes the most common risk factors with known links to the chances of developing cancer:

- age;
- family history;
- exposure to carcinogenic agents such as environmental material, dietary products, alcohol or tobacco smoke;
- viruses;
- hormones.

Some sources can be avoided, others can be controlled, but there are a few which are pre-determined. So the chances of developing any cancer increases with age or if a close relative suffered the same illness.

Benign and malignant tumours

The word tumour means lump and may be used to describe any swelling; it does not mean that the growth is a cancer (a malignant tumour). Most lumps are not cancers and are referred to as benign tumours. Malignant cancers have very definite characteristics, which do not occur in benign tumours. For example:

- malignant tumours tend to be irregular in shape – benign tumours are not;
- malignant tumours invade surrounding tissue – benign tumours do not, they remain contained within the original organ;
- malignant cells break away from the parent tumour and start to grow elsewhere – benign cells do not.

These and other characteristics help doctors to make an informed opinion. But the only true way that a doctor can be sure of the difference is by examining a part of the lump under a microscope to see the pattern of growth and to look at the cells in fine detail. However, the two types do share some features because they are both capable of growing in size beyond that which is comfortable. In this respect both malignant and benign tumours cause pain at the site of the growth, and elsewhere in the body (although tumours that develop in some areas are more likely to cause pain than others). The pain types listed earlier (pages 38–40) can be used to explain and categorise the way tumours behave and have a bearing on the treatment offered. Cancer pain is caused in a number of ways, for example:

- The tumour is pressing on a nerve or a nearby organ. Occasionally this pain is not felt directly at the cancer site because the nerves carry the pain away (referred pain).

- An infection develops at the site of the cancer (or elsewhere) with increased pressure from fluid or pus.

- Scar damage may occur to tissues following surgery.

- Radiotherapy treatment may cause discomfort.

- The cancer may have spread to a secondary site; for example, aching in a limb may be caused by a bone metastasis (a 'break-away' occurrence of the same cancer in the bone).

(There are many organisations specifically targeted to people with cancer and their relatives, see pages 203 and 206 for more details.)

Common causes of non-malignant pain

The illnesses, diseases and syndromes described in the following section have been included because they are some of the most common causes of pain that affect people in the UK. They are grouped in alphabetical order, rather than under body systems, as a convenient way of description. Less common causes have not been mentioned and the order in which they appear has no bearing on the severity, treatments and chances of recovery.

You may wish to start with the entry that explains your own reason for pain (or that of a relative) in more detail, and return to the others at a later stage if appropriate. Use the information about other causes as you wish; however, please try to resist the temptation to fantasise that you are suffering from a number of other conditions – something that can happen all too easily when people are reading about health matters!

A glossary explaining some medical terms can be found on pages 211–212.

Adhesions

Adhesions result from a situation where fibrous tissue forms between two normally unconnected and free-moving surfaces within the body. The condition usually comes about because abnormal healing takes place following a wound (eg abdominal surgery or ulcers) or because tissue has been inflamed due to an infection or damage (eg in a joint). Initially, a large amount of fluid might leak into the cavity, forming a solid mass, which becomes deposited on the sides of nearby structures. The lungs might become connected to the chest wall after pleurisy, or bands form between the stomach, bowel and other abdominal organs following peritonitis. Normally, the layers (called 'fibrin' tissue) would be re-absorbed. But in the case of a severe inflammation, or where repeated attacks have occurred, this does not always happen and the solid mass deposited in this way turns into less absorbable 'fibrous' tissue. The pain occurs when the affected areas tear apart, perhaps after a jerky movement, and because mobility is often restricted.

The history of an infection or surgery in the area is the best indicator as to what might be happening. The sections of tissue that have torn apart then join up together again, thus creating the potential for recurrence. It is sometimes possible to break these lumps down using physiotherapy, but surgery will be necessary to investigate and remove the offending tissue.

Angina

Angina is the name given to pain or 'tightness' that starts in the chest and spreads upwards and outwards, affecting mainly the left side of the upper body. It is most painful in the neck, the jaw and down the left arm. The symptoms can vary in severity from temporary discomfort to a severe, crushing pain that makes the person feel breathless and sick. It occurs when the condition atherosclerosis (furring up of the arteries) prevents sufficient oxygen reaching the heart muscle. The shortage of oxygen is felt when the heart is asked to work harder. It is most likely to occur during increased activity or exertion, when the person is feeling anxious and emotionally stressed, when there is exposure to cold and/or strong wind, or during digestion of a heavy meal when the blood supply is naturally diverted to the stomach.

Occasionally, people experience angina when resting or asleep. Doctors believe this is caused by a spasm (contraction) in the coronary artery that worsens the already poor blood supply. This type of angina is more unstable because the attacks of pain tend to vary in intensity and duration; it should never be ignored.

The first signs of angina-like pain should always be investigated by a doctor, particularly if the feelings of tightness and breathlessness are relieved by resting. Many people treat the early symptoms as indigestion and delay visiting their doctor. It is better to seek early help and be re-assured than to try to 'self-medicate' and allow the disease to progress to a stage where surgery may be necessary or, even worse, a heart attack occurs.

If the symptoms of angina are severe (crushing pain mainly affecting the left-hand side of the body) regard the condition as an emergency. Dial 999 for immediate help, as paramedical teams are trained to give treatment on the spot. The person who is ill should never attempt to drive to hospital.

Angina is not a heart attack but it may be a warning sign that the person is at risk of having one. The doctor will make a diagnosis of angina based on a number of factors: the symptoms describing the pain (what it feels like, how long it lasts, when and how often it occurs); a review of the person's medical history, including any family history; and a physical examination to check heart beat and chest sounds. Various tests are then carried out to help the doctor understand the state of the heart and surrounding arteries. The tests will also rule out conditions with similar signs and symptoms that cause pains in the chest, such as problems in the digestive system or severe anxiety attacks.

Treatment of angina will depend on its severity, and may need to be reviewed if the condition of the heart and surrounding arteries changes. The GP and hospital clinic will check the situation as often as is necessary. The two main courses of treatment are medication and surgery. Drugs (taken when the pain is developing) can swiftly bring the attack under control by relaxing the walls of the arteries and veins, thus allowing an increased flow of blood to the heart and a reduction in the amount of work it has to do to pump the blood around the system. Surgery is now a very effective and successful way of replacing coronary arteries that are blocked. A bypass is created around the blockage by grafting blood vessels from another part of the person's own body, forming a new free-flowing route to the heart. This might be done in as many coronary arteries as necessary (from one to four is common, depending on the level of disease). Another form of surgery, called 'balloon angioplasty', is a relatively new technique used to stretch the coronary artery in many patients with coronary heart disease. The technique is much less invasive than a bypass operation. A long, fine tube is inserted into an artery in the groin and manoeuvred into position at the site of the blocked coronary artery. When correctly placed, the tip of the tube is inflated under high pressure in order to create a wider passage in the artery to allow an increased blood flow. To be valuable, each type of treatment will need to be supported by changes in general lifestyle and some adjustments may have to be made. Recovery rates are good and having angina should not stop a person from living a full and active life. (See pages 202 and 205 for useful addresses.)

Arthritis

Arthritis, in its different forms, is probably one of the commonest reasons for chronic pain. The term refers to any condition affecting joints (limbs or spine) where pain is brought on by inflammation or structural changes. (A similarly painful condition, arthralgia, means pain in the joints where there is no swelling or structural change or indications of arthritis). The most common forms of arthritis are osteoarthritis and rheumatoid arthritits.

Noni's story

Noni has suffered with arthritis for seventeen years in several forms. She has rheumatoid type in her feet, hands and elbows; osteoarthritis in her knees and hips; and ankylosing spondylitis in her spine. Each type can affect her differently on separate days involving, for example, her ability to walk easily or climb stairs. When her spine is hurting she needs to lie down to ease the pain. Altogether Noni finds that her movements are slow.

Noni says that she is reluctant to take too many painkillers as they make her sleepy, but on bad days she does take something as she cannot get out of bed until the tablets have started to work. She finds that the acid in wine makes her joints stiff, as does colder weather. In hot weather inflammation can flare up causing an attack of iritis (see page 211).

For Noni, the three key words that spring to mind in relation to her illness are 'frustration', 'hurt' and 'annoyance' – especially if she is worse on a day when she planned to go out.

In Noni's case the main ways in which her family and friends are affected are that she cannot offer help when it might be needed, and that arrangements have to be cancelled.

The treatment(s) that have worked best for Noni over the years have been a combination of medication and therapies from the following lists:

Prescribed by the general practitioner or hospital consultant
- *Various anti-inflammatory drugs but she has found that she is allergic to all that she has tried*
- *Pain relief – co-codamol works well*
- *Steroid drugs – a short, sharp course is necessary occasionally*
- *Supportive shoes are provided, specially made by the hospital disability services.*

Self-help treatments
- *Multi-vitamin capsules*
- *Evening primrose capsules.*

Complementary therapies
- *None tried.*

Osteoarthritis

This type of arthritis is usually caused by a mechanical failure in the joint, with changes occurring in the articular cartilage (specialised fibrous connective tissue) and bone. The result is a loss of the load-bearing and protective functions of the cartilage, as the shock-absorbing area between the bones cracks, fragments and wears away. Osteoarthritis is a degenerative disease most commonly affecting the hip, knee, spine and finger joints. It is more apparent in middle to old age and found in more women than men. It can be a complication of Perthes' disease, a childhood disorder which caused deformity in the 'growing area' at the top of the thigh bone and affected the weight-bearing part of the hip joint. The first signs of osteoarthritis are gradually increasing pain with swelling and deformity in the affected joint(s). The familiar, lumpy deformities, particularly found in hand joints are caused by outgrowths of cartilage at the edges, which become ossified (like bone). After the early pain subsides (or is treated) more than 50 per cent of people with the condition feel no further pain for several years; however, the deterioration is progressive and irreversible (viewable on X-rays). In severe cases mobility becomes difficult with subsequent symptoms of muscle wasting around the area of the joint.

There are three main causes of osteoarthritis: wear and tear as a result of the ageing process; decline in a joint after an injury or surgical operation (sometimes many years later); and abnormal weight-bearing placed on joints (especially hips and knees) as a result of long-term obesity.

Treatment will usually be a combination of the following options, depending on the probable cause: use of painkilling and non-steroid anti-inflammatory drugs (NSAIDs), which help especially with pain at night and help to reduce stiffness on waking and daytime movements; use of mobility aids to prevent putting too much pressure on the joint but attempting to maintain reasonable levels of activity; and dietary measures to help reduce weight. In advanced cases of cartilage impairment, joint replacement surgery is the best option. As the population that develops osteoarthritis is usually an older one, there are some concerns about taking NSAIDs in the long term – partly because of side effects such as gastric irritation but also because they can impair kidney function. These effects are likely to be more severe in older patients, so you may find that the medical team (especially the physiotherapist) emphasises the importance of using non-drug therapies such as comfort strategies (warmth and gentle movement) which help with function (see page 136). Despite the gloomy prognosis (forecast) about having to live with arthritis for the remainder of your life, the outlook is favourable as most people respond to some form of treatment and the disease is usually slow to develop.

Rheumatoid arthritis

This type of arthritis is caused mainly by chronic inflammation in the synovial linings of joints, tendon sheaths and bursae (sacs of fibrous tissue containing synovial fluid). The synovial lining coats the inside of the joint structure and produces fluid to help lubricate joint movement. The inflammation is not due to an infection in the joint, although the actual triggering reason may not be known. In many cases, the pattern of joint pain is the same on both sides of the body, suggesting a possible single underlying cause. However, not all cases follow this pattern. A genetic disposition is a major factor and the condition is certainly found in family clusters. But as a genetic predisposition alone is not the sole cause, environmental factors probably have a part to play too. The symmetry is one of the symptoms that help doctors diagnose this type of arthritis, together with the fact that the peripheral joints (ie in the hands and feet) are usually affected first and tests show the presence of rheumatoid antibodies in blood serum.

Once the disease is established, it progresses to other joints (for example, wrists, knees, shoulders, ankles and elbows) and repeated attacks of inflammation occur. Most age groups are affected, from mid-twenties to mid-fifties being the most likely age range. Many more women than men are affected (up to a ratio of 4:1). Rheumatoid arthritis is more common in developed countries and, it appears, in people who have moved from a rural to an urban lifestyle. The early signs include swollen joints, which look red and shiny; general stiffness and pain, which is often worse in the mornings, causing limited movement. Sometimes the acute attacks are accompanied by weight loss, a raised temperature and generally feeling unwell. The diagnosis of *carpal tunnel syndrome* (see page 54) may be a forerunner of the disease.

Rheumatoid arthritis lasts for many years with periods of acute attacks usually followed by good periods of remission; in some patients the disease follows a steady downward course resembling a step-like manner. Eventually there is likely to be deformity and loss of movement in the affected joints. Complications of the disease can lead to occasional problems with the lungs (pleurisy) and the eyes (gritty eyes), the connection being the collagen found in connective tissue (see below), which is a constituent of the stiffening material in the transparent jelly of the eye. Anaemia is common (possibly due to the intestinal blood loss caused by the NSAIDs). Once again, despite the dismal description outlined above, the outlook is not totally depressing, as severity of cases vary and about half of people diagnosed continue to lead a relatively normal life. The treatments are similar to those for osteoarthritis, including drug therapy, rest and support for affected joints, always with the aim of maintaining mobility. When an especially acute attack has flared up, steroid drugs may be injected locally into stiff, painful joints bringing short term relief.

Polyarthritis

Polyarthritis is a general term used by some practitioners to describe arthritic-induced inflammation that occurs in several joints, simultaneously. The best example is rheumatoid arthritis but the term can also be used in connection with other forms of arthritis that affect more than one joint.

Psoriatic arthritis

This type is rare and is entirely associated with the skin disorder psoriasis, affecting about one in twenty people with the condition. The problems are caused by inflammation in the affected joints. In most cases the arthritic symptoms are mild with toe and finger joints most commonly painful; the corresponding digits may also show the characteristic pitting signs of psoriasis. In more severe cases any joint might be affected. Treatments are similar to those for rheumatoid arthritis (page 49).

Ankylosing spondylitis

Spondylitis means inflammation in the joints linking the vertebrae in the spinal cord. In 'ankylosing' spondylitis the acute inflammatory period has receded leaving toughened, damaged joints that have become fused together, causing pain and restricted movement of the spine. As the discs and ligaments are replaced by fibrous tissue the spine becomes more rigid. In addition, correct chest expansion is limited because the rib joints are also affected where they connect to the spine. Some chest pain might be felt and patients report tenderness under their heels and pain in their eyes (see effects of collagen, page 49). Early symptoms are indicated by stiffness and pain in the lower back, which tends to be worse in the mornings (conversely, people with a slipped disc feel more pain in the evenings after the stresses of the day). The condition most commonly affects young men and can run in families. Early treatment with anti-inflammatory drugs and physiotherapy is important to help prevent permanent disability.

Reactive arthritis

This is a less common type of arthritis occuring as a secondary illness following an infection elsewhere in the body – for example, colitic arthritis (often associated with a bout of dysentery) and kidney/bladder infections. (See also 'Gout' page 61.)

(See pages 201, 202 and 208 for useful addresses.)

Asthma

Although it is not a true 'pain-producing' illness, asthma, nevertheless, causes much discomfort for people over the years. It presents with four main symptoms – wheezing, breathlessness, cough and chest tightness – and it is the last mentioned symptom that is most likely to be painful, especially in older people. Chronic chest tightness can be very debilitating and may give rise to symptoms similar to angina, so should never be ignored. In addition, asthmatic-like symptoms can also arise in other diseases of the heart or lungs common in older people. These may include chronic bronchitis, emphysema, bronchiectasis and heart failure. (See pages 201 and 207 for useful addresses.)

Back pain

Lower back pain (backache) is one of the oldest problems suffered by humankind, since our ancestors started to walk in an upright position. After several million years of evolutionary development our spines have still not fully adapted to our present posture, from a design more suited to four-footed, horizontal movement. Backache occurs when stress is put on sections of the spine, particularly the lower back and neck areas, where the vertebrae are not supported by the rib cage structure. The lower spine area is very flexible and when too much effort is put into lifting, pulling and various jerky movements, muscles and ligaments become strained. In fact the network of muscles and ligaments is never still, even during sleep. The action of breathing alone causes the whole system to be on the move continually and almost all muscular movements of the main body frame involve the spine in some way.

Backache can have a myriad of causes and is the commonest cause of disability in industrialised nations. However, the most likely reasons tend to be linked to unaccustomed, heavy manual activities such as gardening, moving furniture and (for carers) lifting others. People most at risk tend to come from one of the following categories:

- older people;
- those with a previous weakness;
- people in vulnerable occupations, such as manual and office workers or paramedics;
- people who are very tall or overweight.

Treatments for acute attacks include heat to the area, and painkilling drugs. Current thinking is to keep active, and muscle-relaxing drugs are prescribed.

If there is intense pain and immobility or shooting pains down one or both legs then you should see your doctor as this may indicate a 'prolapsed' or 'slipped' disc which is potentially very serious. This occurs when one or more discs – the rubber-like shock absorbers that sit between most vertebrae in the spine – become dislodged and bulge out of line, pressing on nearby nerves. Intense pain and the inability to move usually necessitates prompt medical assessment to exclude any damage to the collection of nerve roots found at the base of the spine (known as the 'cauda equina' or tail-like structure). Sneezing and coughing can occasionally precipitate such an event. Many people will have some pressure on the nerves surrounding the disc and this gives rise to sciatic-type pain and muscle spasm felt as a 'shooting' or 'stabbing' pain, although some people report a dull ache often in the buttocks. It tends to feel worse when bending and getting up from a seated position or coughing, and the outer leg and foot may feel numb. (In the case of a problem in the neck area, pain will be felt running down the radial nerve in the arms.)

Relatively minor attacks of back pain can be treated with over-the-counter painkillers and rest. Harsher or repeated attacks need medical attention as stronger painkilling drugs can be prescribed. Unless a disc has actually prolapsed, people are no longer recommended to stay immobile, as this can do more harm than good. Physiotherapy often helps and manipulation by an osteopath or chiropractor is sometimes beneficial, but this type of complementary therapy should only be pursued after X-rays have been taken and the treatment is recommended by a registered medical practitioner. Unskilled manipulation could cause serious and permanent spinal injury. In very persistent and painful situations, surgery is recommended to remove a damaged disc. It is also worth emphasising that disc degeneration is a *normal* process. The intervertebral discs start to degenerate and soften from about the mid-twenties onwards. Most people get twinges of discomfort over the years, which usually starts to improve naturally after a few days; more severe cases may take up to six weeks to heal. Recurrent disc injury can become chronic if degeneration is more pronounced.

Angela's story
Angela has had sporadic back pain for many years. Her pain results from an injury which occurred over ten years ago which Angela says flares up every six months or so. For the remainder of the time she is pain-free or feels a dull ache only. She says that when her back is bad it affects everything that she does and when it is very bad it can immobilise her for up to five days at a time. Angela says when her back 'goes' (the household term for her indisposition!) the muscles in her lower back repeatedly go into spasm, locking her into whatever position she happens to be in. The pain is so fierce that she shouts out loud and cries with relief as it subsides. When the pain strikes she sometimes has to

be rescued by her partner from wherever she is stuck, such as the bathroom, or helped from bed and on occasions she has had to be led into the doctor's surgery bent double.

When Angela is off work and alone at home she may end up lying on the floor for days at a time because that is the only place she can rest. This state can make her feel very depressed as she says the pain is terrible. It makes her feel very useless, as though her body is letting her down. The cocktail of prescription drugs which she takes for the inflammation and spasms make her feel very dopey indeed but fortunately she sleeps most of the day; however, they do work as the muscles then relax and restore themselves to a more normal state. Angela finds that lying in pain for a long time is in itself extremely tiring.

The good news is that when her back is not so bad she can get on with things in a relatively normal fashion. The most severe attacks only occur over a few days each year, but the thought of triggering a spasm has made her wary. For example, she cannot sleep in uncomfortable conditions so she now pampers herself and reduces any risk by taking an inflatable bed if she knows that she will be roughing it a bit.

Angela says that her partner and family are extremely distressed by seeing her in so much pain, particularly her mother, as Angela tends to cry a lot with her. Angela's partner has on occasions needed to do everything for her which can be tiring and upsetting for both of them.

For Angela, the three key words that spring to mind in relation to her illness are 'panic', 'fright' and 'debilitating'.

The treatment(s) that have worked best for Angela over the years have been a combination of medication and therapies from the following lists:

Prescribed by the general practitioner or hospital consultant
- *Muscle relaxant (diazepam) – used to relax the muscle spasms*
- *Non-steroidal anti-inflammatory/analgesic (diclofenac) – used for pain relief and to help reduce inflammation when her acute musculo-skeletal condition is acute*
- *Pain relief (solpadol) – taken short term in high dosages to relieve severe pain.*

Self-help treatments
- *Lying on her back on the floor with knees up, rocking gently from side-to-side which helps to calm the spasm.*
- *Sleeping on the floor for a few days, staying very still.*
- *Swimming a lot when her back is well she finds is a good way of strengthening the muscles that need to step in and take over when her back 'goes'.*

Complementary therapies
- *Arnica 'shock' pills help when the pain is very bad and Angela gets worked up and panicky and cries a lot.*

Angela says that she has never attended a pain clinic.

People who suffer chronic problems may need to consider other measures, described more fully in Chapter Three and Four. (See also Arthritis pages 46–50, Lumbago page 65, Osteoporosis page 70, and Sciatica page 75. Page 201 gives a list of useful addresses.)

Bell's palsy

Bell's palsy is relatively uncommon in that it affects less than one in 1,000 people annually but its sudden appearance is worrying. The most obvious symptom is drooping of the face caused by paralysis of the facial nerve, triggered by inflammation. The whole of one side of the face is affected with weakness in the muscles from the forehead down to the chin; the mouth hangs down, the tongue movement is impaired and the eyelid cannot be closed. Paralysis does not occur elsewhere in the body. The person is likely to feel pain and discomfort around the area, especially in the region of the ear. The paralysis usually improves after a few weeks; however, there may be damage to the eye and permanent facial weakness or paralysis may persist. It is important to close the eye manually with a gentle action at regular intervals to help keep it moist, perhaps aided by saline eye drops. A course of steroid injections may be given if discomfort and paralysis continue.

Carpal tunnel syndrome

This is a condition where a nerve leading to the hand becomes compressed in an aperture in the wrist, called the carpal tunnel, the passageway that gives protection to the tendons that flex the fingers. The problem occurs because pressure builds up over the years as the tendons thicken, together with damage to the tunnel caused by other disorders such as arthritis in the wrist joint. The symptoms of persistent pain, tingling and numbness in the area around the thumb and first two fingers are often worse at night or when the hand is very warm. Eventually some loss of movement, with chronic muscle weakness and wastage, occurs and the pain may progress up the arm. The disorder is most common in people who have spent many years using a keyboard as a typist or a pianist. Treatment relies on painkilling drugs and restriction of movement with a splint. In severe cases steroid injections may help, or surgery may be needed to relieve pressure on the nerve.

Cerebral palsy

Cerebral palsy is an example of a condition that is present at birth causing permanent damage to an area of the brain. In the majority of cases the abnormality dates from the period the baby is in the womb such as a malformation of the brain or as the result of an infection affecting the unborn baby's brain. In a smaller number of cases the disability results from a birth injury or shortage of oxygen to the baby's brain during a difficult labour. It is characterised by impaired muscle control with painful muscle spasms. The severity and range of disability varies, depending on the site of the original damage. The results of such brain defects are likely to cause chronic discomfort over many years. All treatment is aimed at controlling and improving any symptoms to achieve an active and fulfilling lifestyle.

Collagen diseases

Linked to arthritis (pages 46–50) are a number of conditions sometimes described collectively as 'collagen diseases' because they all involve connective tissue. These diseases are rare but they may flare up anywhere in the body, as collagen is the main component of connective tissue, an essential part of every structure. The main organs where inflammation could occur include the eyes, skin, heart, lungs and kidneys, as well as joint involvement. Examples of collagen disease include systemic sclerosis, systemic lupus and polyarthritis, (see also Polymyalgia rheumatica page 72).

Constipation

Chronic constipation is mainly found in older people where the bowel movements have become sluggish, primarily due to lax muscles, and made worse by poor diet and an increasing use of drugs that have a constipating effect. Other causes include cancer of the bowel, bowel obstruction and reluctance to pass a motion because tears and fissures in the passage around the anus make bowel movements very painful. The constipation itself can also cause intense abdominal pain. Treatment includes attention to an appropriate diet, extra fluids and careful use of laxative medicines and suppositories to help regulate bowel action. It is also important to be aware that a daily bowel movement is not essential and for some people may not be their normal pattern (see also Haemorrhoids, page 62).

Crohn's disease (ileitis)

This chronic disorder is caused by inflammation in the ileum, the lower part of the small bowel. The intestine wall becomes thickened, fluid accumulates in the tissues, ulcers develop and an infection sets in. In extreme cases the ulcers penetrate the bowel wall leading potentially to peritonitis. Where the tissue has healed scarring may produce constricting rings in the bowel. Once established, the condition can become a lifelong problem with chronic diarrhoea and repeated attacks of severe abdominal pain. The exact cause is unknown but it does run in families. Treatment includes careful attention to diet, anti-diarrhoeal medication to ease the symptoms, which should also reduce the attacks of abdominal cramp. Long-term care may be helped by occasional steroid therapy and possible surgery to remove areas of damaged bowel. (See page 207 for useful addresses.)

Dental problems

Dental pain (toothache) is a classic example of acute pain, when inflammation builds up in the pulp cavity at the heart of the tooth. If the pulp becomes infected, because food material seeps inwards through a crack in the tooth, pus can develop, forming an abscess. In such a small space the pressure on the nerve can cause extreme pain. Less acute, but often very sharp, dental pain can occur where areas of enamel have become chipped or worn away, leaving the dentine layer beneath unprotected. Loss of enamel can occur through trauma or because the gums have receded, exposing the dentine. This type of pain is triggered more often by eating hot, cold or sweet foods and is often eased by using special toothpaste designed to reduce sensitivity. Expert dental treatment is always necessary to repair a cavity in a tooth and an antibiotic would be given if an abscess had developed. Immediate pain relief can be achieved with painkillers and an old-fashioned, but still effective, remedy is to bite on a piece of cotton wool soaked in essential oil of cloves; the oil penetrates into the crack and has a soothing, numbing action.

Diabetic neuropathy

Diabetes is a huge topic in itself; however, diabetic neuropathy is particularly relevant when discussing pain. It is a complication of diabetes that may develop after many years, affecting the nerve pathways, either singly or generally. The symptoms include pain, tingling and numbness in hands and feet, caused by damage to the sensory nerves that lead to these areas. The presence of a neuropathic condition makes the foot less sensitive to pain and temperature, but the reduced sensation (a feeling of walking on cotton wool or gravel) makes people with diabetes more prone to foot injuries and infections. Daily foot care and checking bathwater temperature are sensible precautions to take. (See pages 204 and 208 for useful addresses.)

Diverticulitis

'Diverticula' is the name given to the pouches that line the walls of the gut. Faecal matter gets pushed into the pouches and can become trapped and infected. Many people by middle age have extended diverticular pouches, but most drain easily and cause no complications; however, in the minority of people symptoms can arise giving much discomfort caused by trapped wind and a distended abdomen. The pain is felt particularly as a persistent ache in the lower left abdomen. Immediate treatment, such as a warm hot-water bottle and rest will help to improve acute symptoms, possibly with a course of antibiotics to deal with the infection. Long-term care should focus on improving the fibre content of the diet. (See pages 202 and 206 for useful addresses.)

Dyspepsia (indigestion)

Indigestion, to give dyspepsia its common name, usually results from eating too much or too rich a diet. It causes acute pain in the upper middle part of the abdomen, often accompanied by wind and distension. Chronic indigestion causes severe discomfort for some people over the years, often with symptoms of acid and food regurgitation into the oesophagus (gullet) and up to the throat causing heartburn and nausea. Attention to diet is the best treatment but medical advice should be sought if the problem persists because it may be a sign that stomach ulcers are present. Sometimes the pain can be felt in the shoulderblade area (an example of referred pain).

Endometriosis

Endometriosis is a disorder of the female reproductive system where cells normally found in the lining of the uterus (womb) grow in other, abnormal places in the pelvic area. The lining of the Fallopian tubes, in the ovaries and on the pelvic wall behind the uterus are prime sites. The displaced tissue behaves like uterine tissue causing considerable pain and dull aching in the lower back and abdominal areas, which becomes worse at the time of menstruation. Pain can also occur during sexual intercourse. The cause is unknown and can be felt throughout the fertile years. Treatment for less severe cases would be similar to that for typical menstrual pain: painkilling drugs and adopting a warm, comfortable position. More severe cases may respond to hormone treatment, or surgery to remove the patches might be considered. (See page 207 for useful addresses.)

Fibromyalgia

This is a chronic syndrome which is characterised by widespread musculo-skeletal pain and multiple localised 'tender points' such as neck, spine, shoulders and hips, where hard nodular lumps may sometimes be felt. There is chronic pain with acute flare ups and disturbed sleep. The cause is still unknown but is thought to be related to previous infection or trauma and may be exacerbated in someone whose pain threshhold feels lower, especially in damp conditions. *Bandolier's Little Book of Pain* says that '10% of the population may have widespread pain, with more folk in their 60s …' Warmth from a suitable heat source such as a wheat bag, or using a TENS machine, together with painkillers, is the best home treatment.

Frozen shoulder (periarthritis)

Pain from a 'frozen' shoulder tends to affect people from middle age onwards. Limited movement in the shoulder joint makes it impossible to lift the affected arm upwards or backwards or to perform the full range of normal joint action. Inflammation in the surrounding area causes pain and stiffness, increasing the discomfort, which is usually worse at night. There are three main reasons why the condition commonly causes joint pain – injury, repetitive movement or unaccustomed and (strenuous) exercise – but an obvious trigger cannot always be identified.

Frozen shoulder is also associated with the term *painful arc syndrome,* where the person is unable to move their arm sideways. Similar problems can affect other joints, which, over the years, have been given descriptive names such as *tennis* or *golfers' elbow.* Treatment with painkilling and anti-inflammatory drugs, resting the limb and physiotherapy, is important to prevent permanent damage to these various joints. Recovery is gradual and may take up to two years.

Gall stones

Solid material in the gall bladder and the bile ducts forms into gravel or pebble-like masses (calculi). The 'stones' build up over the years following repeated attacks of inflammation in the gall bladder, known as chronic cholecystitis. The problem is relatively common, affecting about one in ten people and rising to one in five after middle age. If the stones remain dormant symptoms are few and may be detected only by X-ray examination; however, people with painful symptoms usually find the discomfort starts after eating a meal rich in fat. As the digestive process commences pain is felt in the upper abdominal region, with wind and a bloated feeling. In more severe cases the pain progresses from the abdomen through to the shoulder blade, known as referred pain. The pain is most relentless when the stones move in the bile duct, often accompanied by nausea and vomiting.

Complications, including jaundice and inflammation to the pancreas, may develop if the output of bile juices from the gall bladder is blocked. Immediate treatment includes taking painkilling drugs. Drinking warm water and resting also helps until the acute phase of the cholecystitis passes. If the symptoms worsen, a doctor should be consulted as moving stones can cause excruciating pain. In the long term, changes should be made to the diet to reduce the fat content. Other options, such as surgery or stone-dissolving medication or disintegration by powerful sound waves may be considered.

Glaucoma

Glaucoma is more commonly found in older people, especially women, and it can present as an acute or chronic disorder. Both types are serious and delay in seeking treatment could lead to irreversible damage and possible blindness. (See page 206 for useful addresses.)

Acute glaucoma

An acute attack must be treated as an emergency, because the eye is unlikely to recover independently. Symptoms in an acute attack cause severe pain in and around the eye; blurred and disturbed vision; the pain is often intense enough to cause vomiting. Early warnings signs may start with discomfort, hazy vision and rainbow haloes around lights; these short-lived attacks tend to become stronger, so medical help should be sought before the full-blown phase sets in. The problem is caused by a blockage in the channel running around the edge of the inside of the iris (the coloured part of the eye which contracts to regulate light into the pupil). Fluid cannot drain away from the area between the lens and the cornea and pressure swiftly builds up in the eyeball. Eventually, pressure on the nerve fibres at the back of the eye could damage the eyesight. The effects of the blockage become worse as the iris tries to dilate because of reduction in light levels, and as an automatic reaction to additional excitement (or nervousness). Treatment is aimed at reducing the effects of the pressure, with eye drops to make the pupil smaller and a painkilling injection. Hospitalisation may be necessary.

Chronic glaucoma

The chronic version should also be dealt with quickly, once any symptoms are felt, as vision in both eyes can be affected. This type almost always occurs in older people and a family history is common. The great problem is that there are few noticeable warning signs. Slowly, over a longish period (months or even years), sight is reduced at the edges of the visual field. There is no obvious pain in chronic glaucoma. Adjustments are made to the declining vision and actual loss may not be reported until a fair degree of incurable damage is present. In the chronic version, excess pressure builds up in the eyeball very slowly and is thought to be due to a gradual deterioration in the circulatory mechanism, which takes fluid away from the eye – probably due to an increasing failure in the circulatory system in general. Treatment again is aimed at reducing pressure in the eyeball, so eye drops are inserted regularly and a special drainage operation may be considered.

Gout

Gout is an illness that occurs primarily in men, at any age, but increasingly as they get older. Women are rarely affected and if so it is usually post-menopausal. Gout is one of the most common forms of joint disease and is not, as cartoon characters suggest, a result of overindulgence in rich foods! A sudden, very painful attack, commonly in the big toe joint, is the most obvious symptom, accompanied by signs of acute inflammation. Other joints – knees, ankles and wrists – may also be affected and stones may form in the kidneys. The inflammation is caused when crystals of uric acid (a product of urine metabolism) are deposited in the joint area and the surrounding tissue becomes tender. If the condition is not treated swiftly the person often feels very ill. Once established the condition tends to become chronic with no absolute cure; acute attacks are likely to flare up at variable intervals. Repeated attacks lead eventually to arthritic joint problems and other complications include high blood pressure and heart disease. The true cause is unknown, other than a probable genetic weakness in fully eliminating the by-products of urine from the body. Gout can be controlled very successfully by drug treatment and avoiding certain foods which have triggered past attacks.

Dennis and Louise
Louise's husband Dennis suffers from gout. She describes his first attack:

'We'd been so busy with the house move and everything. Then we went off to France on holiday and while we were there his foot swelled up. It went all hot and red, and was just so painful. I thought gout only happened to people who ate and drank too much, but the doctor said it's nothing to do with that really and he shouldn't be embarrassed. It completely ruined our holiday though.'

Haemorrhoids (piles)

Haemorrhoids are the distended varicose veins in the area close to the anus, which can develop inside and outside the back passage. The enlarged veins tend to get worse over the years and result from over-straining to pass motions. The piles frequently bleed and can be very painful when swollen and inflamed. Warm baths and a hot flannel pressed on the area help to relieve the pain and soothing, local anaesthetic creams and suppositories are readily available from pharmacies and most supermarkets. In severe conditions surgery would be considered to remove the excess tissue. (See also Constipation, page 56).

Hernia

A hernia is the collective name given to a protrusion of various abdominal organs (usually the gut) through a gap in the structure of the abdominal wall. The common name is a 'rupture'. A particular hernia is then named according to the site where it occurs:

- **Inguinal hernia** This is the most common type and found more commonly in men. It shows as a bulge above the groin crease and the protrusion frequently slips into the scrotum where it can appear as a very large lump.

- **Femoral hernia** This type is more common in women and appears as a much smaller lump, usually just below the groin crease.

- **Umbilical hernia** This type is most common in babies at the site of the umbilical cord.

- **Midline hernia** This type generally occurs in women who have had multiple births. The weakened muscle wall of the abdomen bulges when sitting up from a lying position.

- **Hiatus hernia** This type is caused by a bulging of the stomach up through the diaphragm at the weakest point where the oesophagus (gullet) enters the abdomen. The hernia is not visible from the outside.

- **Incisional hernia** This type occurs at the site of a previous wound or surgery, particularly when the lower tissues have not knitted together well.

The symptoms for most types are similar – there is pain and discomfort at the site where the bulge occurs, which is more obvious when straining or coughing. A hernia may slip in and out of the abdominal wall and may be pushed back gently by hand, but cannot be permanently cured without surgical repair. A hernia that becomes over swollen may strangulate, cutting off the blood supply to the area. This is very painful and is a serious medical emergency.

Hip degeneration

The hip joint is one of the most common sites associated with chronic pain, especially in the older age group. The problem is most likely to be due to degeneration of the ball and socket structure of the joint, caused by osteoarthritis (see page 47). In a small minority of people (mainly women) the breakdown could be the result of a lifetime's walking with an un-repaired congenital dislocated hip joint (a unilateral birth defect). Hip replacement surgery is now a standard procedure, relieving pain and restoring mobility for many people.

Intermittent claudication

(See Peripheral vascular disease, page 72)

Irritable bowel syndrome (IBS)

This disorder (also known as spastic colon) commonly starts in younger people and may persist for many years into older age. It induces urgent diarrhoea especially after meals, often accompanied by strong, colicky pain felt most in the lower left-hand side of the abdomen (above the colon). Other symptoms include feelings of tension, anxiety and depression, which can be instrumental in causing the muscles of the bowel to over react. Treatments include attention to diet, possibly supplemented with medication or bran to bulk out the diet, and measures to identify and reduce raised stress levels. (See page 210 for useful addresses.)

Richard's story
Richard has suffered from IBS for as long as he can remember – certainly since he was a university student. The problem is not constant, sometimes he goes for many months without symptoms. Then everything flares up again. He is conscious of

a dull pain, usually on the lower right side of his abdomen, but sometimes this is accompanied by sharp or stabbing pains at the same site or elsewhere. Pain under the ribcage is not uncommon too.

Usually, Richard is able to get on with life in the normal way despite the pain. It is unusual for it to be severe enough to make him need to stop or lie down. Although it might make it hard for him to get to sleep sometimes, it doesn't wake him up. More troublesome are the accompanying symptoms of needing to get to the toilet in a hurry, and the uncomfortable sensation of trapped wind (sometimes leading to acute embarrassment when the trap is sprung).

While still in his thirties, Richard was advised to eat a high fibre diet with extra bran, but unfortunately the bran seemed to make things worse in his case. He tries to eat plenty of fresh vegetables but too much fruit can result in acidity which can add to the problems. Richard has tried to identify dietary triggers (but failed), though he does realise that stress and lack of sleep make the problem worse.

Prescribed medications that have helped over the years include various different antispasmodic preparations (alverine, mebeverine, peppermint oil).

Self-help measures include attempting to eat a balanced diet, and drinking plenty of water. However, Richard has been unable to give up drinking tea or coffee.

He has also tried one complementary therapy – reflexology. He says he enjoyed the regular appointments for about a year, but ended up feeling that they didn't actually do anything for the IBS.

Now, Richard is not receiving any treatment (and has not done for some years). He accepts that abdominal pain and the associated symptoms are a fact of life, and does his best to live a normal life around them.

Ischaemia

The medical term means lack of the blood supply to any body part, due to a number of causes that, effectively, obstruct an artery: contraction, constriction, muscle spasm and blocking by a blood clot are the most common reasons. A stroke (see page 77) is a severe (and sometimes permanent) result of cerebral ischaemia. A migraine (see below) is a temporary form. One of the main symptoms is pain in the organ beyond the obstruction and always requires some form of treatment. For example, a person suffering with angina pain (see page 44) could bring about immediate relief by using a drug that relaxes the artery walls; a person with leg cramps (see page 72) would need to rest.

Lumbago

This term means severe pain in the lower back area (lumbar region) usually triggered by lifting a heavy object or bending over (see Back pain, page 51). The pain can be very severe and might immobilise the person in the stooping position until it eases. It gradually improves with rest but could be an early sign of a slipped or prolapsed disc, as the pain is due primarily to pressure on the sciatic nerve. Investigations may be necessary if the problem returns.

Migraine

It is a rare person who has not at some time suffered a severe headache, perhaps as a symptom of an illness or after a heavy bout of drinking alcohol. This type of headache is transient, improves after a short while and usually has a known cause. Migraine is less easy to identify with an obvious cause and comes under the general heading 'benign recurring headaches'. (The term 'benign' is used when describing this type of headache to indicate that the cause is not malignant or cancerous in nature – it does not mean that a migraine is a small problem!) Headaches, including migraine and those brought on by muscular pain from the neck, account for the majority of reasons why people visit their doctor. An estimated 5 per cent of the population suffer from migraine; women are more prone than men and it tends to run in families.

Typical symptoms in the severest form (classic migraine) include many or all of the following, starting with early warning signs that indicate a migraine is pending:

- visual disturbances, usually seen in both eyes;
- numbness, tingling and/or weakness in part of the face, a hand or a leg, which may spread or move around;
- feelings of confusion and dizziness;

- speech difficulties;

- photophobia (dislike of light).

These initial symptoms wear off and are soon followed by the relentless throbbing headache, typical of a migraine. The pain in the head may be one-sided and tends to be felt on the opposite side to the body symptoms. Nausea and vomiting are often present. In the less harsh form, called a common migraine, the headache only is present.

Migraine attacks vary greatly with individual people, appearing regularly or infrequently, with symptoms lasting several hours to a few days. It is often associated with the menstrual cycle. The initial symptoms are caused by a sudden constricting of the arteries leading to one side of the head (see ischaemia above). The headache occurs at the stage where the blood vessels re-expand allowing a large flow of blood back into the area. The exact reason why this action occurs is unknown. Many activators are blamed and different people can often pinpoint personal triggers. Common agents include stress, emotional upsets, overwork, flashing (strobing) lights and certain food combinations or drugs. The migraine is most likely to start a short while after the triggering event has passed, rather than immediately at the time. (See page 206 for useful addresses.)

Anya's story

Anya has lived with migraine attacks for 38 years, a long time to live with the uncertainty of never knowing when it's going to attack again. She says that she has no signs that a migraine is coming. One of her worst fears is being caught out by the inconvenience and not being able to prepare. At times, she says, it is a complete 'dread' almost waiting for a migraine to strike when she least needs it such as during a holiday or special evening out. Her migraines can also affect her capacity to drive.

For Anya, the three key words that spring to mind in relation to her illness are 'inconvenience', 'frustration' and 'disbelief'.

Anya says that her migraines affect her work colleagues mainly, as she has to take two pain-relieving tablets and sit with her eyes closed for up to forty minutes until her vision has cleared. (The tablet that works best for her is Migraleve, a compound of various analgesic drugs.)

The treatment that has worked best for Anya over the years has been a self-help version only:

- *Pain relieving tablets, which Anya keeps in a her handbag at all times.*

She has not tried any complementary therapies – or had drugs prescribed by a general practitioner or hospital consultant.

Neither has Anya attended a pain clinic because, apart from the inconvenience, she feels she has the situation under control.

Motor neurone disease

This disease affects the central nervous system (brain and spinal cord area) gradually destroying the nerves that carry messages to and from the muscles. The damage occurs in the neurone (nerve cell) part of the nerve structure. The symptoms of weakness are felt first in the outer limbs – legs, feet or hands and, because of its progressive nature, migrate upwards to the essential, core muscles of the body. As the muscles waste away they become stiff and painful with spastic-like spasms; muscle twitching is common. All muscles are eventually involved thus affecting the ability to swallow, breathe and speak. The true cause is unknown but viral links are suspected. The lifespan of the person may be limited from onset of symptoms to severe disability and death. There is no cure for motor neurone disease so treatments are aimed at reducing the distressing symptoms. (See page 206 for useful address.)

Multiple sclerosis

Sometimes called disseminated sclerosis, this disease again affects the function of the central nervous system. Hardened patches develop irregularly (disseminated means spread out) in the insulating sheath structure surrounding individual nerve cells. The sheath substance initially breaks down and is absorbed, leaving areas where the nerve fibre is bare. Eventually this is replaced by connective-type tissue in a much denser mass than would normally be present. The nerves are unable to function properly causing disturbance in sight, sensation and movement. Pain accompanies these various disabilities, behind the eyes and during efforts to coordinate degenerating muscle control. The disorder is usually progressively disabling over a course of many years. The cause is unknown but is linked to possible viral action; there is no cure. Treatment programmes, using drugs, diet and physiotherapy, are designed to alleviate symptoms. (See page 207 for useful addresses.)

Myalgia

The general term means pain in a muscle, it is therefore used as a description in many disorders. Specifically, the illness known as 'myalgic encephalomyelitis (ME)', is a disease that causes muscle weakness, extreme tiredness and pain brought on by minimal exertion. The debilitating symptoms can last for many months and, although the signs resemble those caused by similar viral infections, a related virus has yet to be identified. The treatment focuses mainly on rest and relieving the painful symptoms. (See page 201 for useful address.)

Neck injuries and pain

Neck injuries, like back pain, tend to be caused by undue stress being put on sections of the upper spine. The most common reason is accidental injury which could damage any of the structural parts making up the neck: muscles, spinal cord, vertebrae, windpipe, oesophagus, nerves and blood vessels all run through this area. Because of the vulnerability of these vital systems, professionally trained paramedics should treat any suspected injury to the neck. Mishandling of a casualty, for example; following a road accident, could cause permanent paralysis and even death. (See also Whiplash; page 82). Neck pain may also start up, quite suddenly, for non-accidental reasons. The most likely cause is a twisted, strained muscle, which eases with rest and painkilling drugs. However, the cause might be due to viral or bacterial action. If the stiffness is accompanied by other symptoms indicating an infection in the brain or spinal cord; such as a raised temperature, severe headache, vomiting, difficulty bending the neck, a dislike of light and paralysis, medical advice should be sought immediately to rule out (or treat urgently) the serious illness, meningitis. Although meningitis is usually thought of as a young person's disease it can affect people of any age, so symptoms similar to those listed above should never be treated lightly. The pain resulting from a milder viral illness will subside after a few days.

Neuralgia

This is the name given to any pain that originates from an inflamed, irritated or compressed nerve and is usually felt along the whole of the nerve pathway, not only at the site of the problem. This discomfort may affect any nerve in the body and the resulting pain tends to be felt in two different ways: as a persistent, dull ache which can be very severe, such as in shingles (see page 75) or as a sharp, intense spurt, which is felt when the nerve is activated. The different types, although brought about for different reasons, tend to share similar symptoms. A fractured bone or slipped disc (see page 51) may compress the nerve causing excruciating, knife-like pain to the point where it causes immobility, or it can be felt as an ever-present niggle. Irritation of a sensory nerve, such as that to the side of the face can cause a condition known as *trigeminal neuralgia,* named after the trigeminal nerve that feeds the area covering the lips, gums, cheek and temple. Very severe pain is felt when abnormal electrical bursts are discharged along the nerve. The attacks are brief, lasting only a few seconds and may be sporadic in nature over many years. The pain could be set off by a number of triggers, such as, cold, pressure, certain facial movements, dental problems and atheroma (fatty arterial plaques) may play a part in older people. Painkilling drugs help to alleviate discomfort and in severe cases the trigeminal nerve can be destroyed by injection or surgery; occasionally it clears up spontaneously. If the trigger can be isolated, then avoidance is an obvious way of preventing attacks. (See page 209 for useful addresses.)

Neurofibroma

A neurofibroma is a benign (non-malignant) tumour that grows in a nerve pathway. The tumour is most commonly found close to the skin surface and is relatively symptomless, until it grows large enough to cause pain through pressure on the nerve. A related disorder, called 'neurofibromatosis' is a genetic disease producing multiple lumps all over the body. The lumps are caused by excessive growth of nerve fibres.

Osteoarthritis

(See page 47)

Osteomyelitis

Osteomyelitis is a bacterial infection of bones that starts with severe and sudden pain, fever, tenderness and swelling in the affected area, usually a limb. The condition is most likely to be found in younger people but can affect any age group. Antibiotic treatment is given in the acute phase, but if the infection is severe or becomes well established it can be difficult to cure. It can arise following an infected wound or more generally because of bacteria in the bloodstream. In the chronic phase, the disease may spread to adjacent bones.

Osteoporosis

Osteoporosis is the medical name for weakening of the bones. The disorder is found most commonly in post-menopausal women but can affect other age groups and men. The condition shows up on X-ray as a reduced mass of normal bone, due to excessive resorption of the bone (ie the bone is absorbed back into itself), rather than as a decrease in new bone formation. The quality of the remaining bone is adequate, it is the quantity that becomes reduced. After the menopause women naturally discontinue their production of the hormone oestrogen, which is then linked to loss of calcium and resulting changes in bone structure. As a consequence of this inevitable process, women lose approximately one per cent of their bone mass each year unless HRT (hormone replacement therapy) is being taken. Men are much less affected. Research has found that the condition is more severe in white women than black women; in people who smoke; in people who are very thin and people who have exercised less over the years; in people who have taken prolonged courses of steroid drugs and where there is a family history. The thinning of the bones leads to some obvious signs, for example, where compression of the bones in the vertebrae cause a loss of height, curvature in the upper spine (dowager's or widow's hump) and backache in the lower, lumbar region. All weakened areas in the bones are vulnerable to fracturing: minor cracks might result from everyday knocks, while major breaks, commonly to the arms, shoulder bone, thighs or pelvis, might result from accidental falls.

Osteoporosis itself gives no true symptoms other than backache, but the after effects of a related injury could be very painful. The condition is permanent and progressive, and treatment is aimed at relieving symptoms or dealing with fractures. Hormone replacement therapy can be a valuable preventive measure in younger women but this course of action must be discussed thoroughly with a doctor and weighed against other drawbacks. Replacement calcium (with vitamin D to aid absorption) can be taken to supplement dietary amounts to help maintain levels of bone calcium but it is not possible to increase significantly the levels as people age (after about 35 years). (See page 207 for useful address.)

Paget's disease

This disease causes a progressive thickening and softening of the bones, mainly affecting the skull, spine, pelvis and legs, in people of middle age and over. It is one of the commonest bone diseases in the world with many hundreds of thousands of people in the UK affected (about 600,000 people in England). The symptoms include dull, persistent pain that is worse when activity is increased. The cause of the disease is unknown and there is no cure. Treatment, such as taking painkilling drugs, is aimed at reducing the unpleasant effects of the disease. Supplements of calcium, vitamins and hormones may also be recommended. (See page 207 for useful address.)

Parkinson's disease

Parkinson's disease affects the central nervous system, causing marked muscular stiffness and tremors. These become progressively more unpleasant as the illness worsens. This disease is found more commonly in men than women, and is rare in people under the age of fifty. It is estimated that about ten thousand people develop Parkinson's disease in the UK every year. In the early stages the progression is usually gradual, with little trouble from symptoms. In the later stages tremors in the limbs and involuntary head nodding (while the person is awake) become more common. Limbs stiffen and become resistant to movement, causing considerable pain. As the muscles of the face lose flexibility, the person assumes a characteristic, unblinking expression. Deterioration generally occurs slowly over many years but in some people the degeneration process is much swifter. The symptoms are caused by a deficiency in a brain chemical called dopamine. Researchers do not yet know why this reduction occurs; however, there may be links to smoking and genetics. Parkinsonism (Parkinson-like symptoms) can be triggered by side effects of drugs and is commonly seen in older people with poor circulation to the brain caused by atheroma (see page 211). (See page 208 for useful addresses.)

Peripheral vascular disease (leg cramps)

Peripheral vascular disease occurs as a direct result of the 'hardening' and 'furring up' of the arteries (atherosclerosis), and causes unpleasant leg cramps when increased activity calls for additional oxygen to the muscles. When the blood supply is reduced, exercise causes severe pain, which stops at rest – a condition known as *intermittent claudication.* If the blood supply is very poor, the pain can occur even when the person is resting. If painful leg cramps are occurring, a medical check should be made because high blood pressure and diabetes are known causes. People with severe peripheral vascular disease are at risk of developing leg ulcers, so care must be taken to prevent skin damage from broken toenails or from knocking against furniture.

Treatment of peripheral vascular disease is given in several ways, including:

- exercise and maintaining activity levels;
- stopping aggravation factors (such as smoking);
- medication;
- surgical bypass;
- stretching of the artery at the site of the blockage.

Polymyalgia rheumatica

This disorder is one of the group of 'collagen' diseases, similar to arthritis. Collagen is a fibrous structure found in bone cartilage and all other connective tissues. The condition produces stiffness in the shoulders, particularly first thing in the morning. Treatment with suitable drugs brings about effective relief.

Raynaud's syndrome

This is a circulatory illness affecting the extremities of people who are unduly sensitive to cold conditions. The hands, fingers and feet turn white and then blue and become numb (if allowed); the skin becomes red as the circulation is restored. The attack lasts for about 15 minutes provided the affected parts are re-warmed. The reduced circulation is caused by a contraction of the arteries supplying the area and may be triggered by the pressure created by gripping a heavy object. Other causes include industrial effects (for example, handling heavy power machinery); side effects of certain drugs; smoking; inflammation of arteries; and nerve paralysis. The main preventive measure is keeping the limbs warm and avoiding triggering an attack brought on by vibration or constriction. Prescribed drugs can alleviate symptoms in more severe cases.

Renal colic (kidney, bladder and ureter stones)

Stones which form in the kidneys (called calculi) are similar in make up to stones that form in other organs, such as the gall bladder (see page 59). They develop from excess salts in the bloodstream, which then form crystals in the urine and settle in one or both kidneys. Occasionally they can form after an infection in the urinary tract, especially if a blockage hinders or obstructs the flow of urine. Often the person does not drink sufficient fluids to flush through the system and problems may arise following a prolonged period of immobility. The stones can resemble small pieces of gravel, or be several in number, or there could be a single stone that grows to a relatively large size. The stones grow to fit the internal space of the organ. In the kidney they will always be irregular in shape. Stones that grow in the ureters (the tubes that carry urine from the kidneys to the bladder) tend to be smoother and elongated in shape; those that develop in the relatively open space in the bladder are usually larger, smoother and more pebble-like. Gravel can develop over a few weeks but large stones take years to grow.

As long as the stones remain dormant they rarely cause any symptoms. The trouble starts when a stone begins to move out of the kidney and migrates down the urinary tract. Because of its rough edges the stone tears the lining of the urinary tract as it moves, causing extreme pain. The level of pain from stones moving from the ureters and the bladder is usually lower. The first sign of pain from a kidney stone starts in the middle of the back; it then spreads to the front of the abdomen and down into the sexual organs. The pain builds to a peak, lasts for about a minute, subsides for a few minutes and then repeats the pattern. There is usually pain on passing urine and blood may be seen in the water. Annually, about one person in two thousand in the UK will have kidney stones. They are also more common in certain geographical areas where the natural water is harder and contains particular minerals that trigger stone formation. The immediate treatment involves strong, pain-killing injections, as the acute phase is very painful. Subsequent treatment depends on the state of the stones. There are several possible options including surgical removal via a 'keyhole' slit, or disintegration using powerful sound waves. The kidney may have to be removed if it has been very badly damaged.

Repetitive strain injury

The medical term for this condition is 'tenosynovitis' and, as its common name suggests, repeated movement of some description causes the injury. The pain occurs because the sheath of tissue surrounding a tendon (the fibrous cord that attaches muscle to bone) becomes inflamed at the point where the tendon passes over a joint. The wrist, shoulder and ankle are common sites. In addition to the pain felt on movement, the joint or tendon will often also creak. The disorder quickly descends from the acute stage of inflammation into a chronic state that may last several years, especially if overuse of the joint or tendon area continues. The condition often affects people who use a typewriter or computer keyboard very regularly and if their income relies on this type of work having to rest the strained area for long periods or reducing the repetitive movement are not always straightforward options. Painkilling drugs help to ease the discomfort and immobilising the joint, whenever convenient, aids the healing process. Some cases may benefit from a course of physiotherapy. Preventative measures include changing working practice to adopt a less straining movement and using specially (ergonomically) designed furniture. The injury is likely to recur unless the contributing conditions are altered.

Rheumatism

This word is now obsolete in medical terms, with no defined meaning, but is still commonly used to describe any pain felt in the limbs and spine.

Rheumatoid arthritis

(See page 48)

Scoliosis

The term means a sideways curvature of the spine and may be the result of a birth defect such as cerebral palsy, or an illness such as poliomyelitis, or a structural disorder which affects the spine during the growing period. In later life a curvature may develop as a result of attempting to ease severe pain caused by a spinal problem, such as a slipped disc (see below). The initial treatment in childhood would have included some type of support and/or surgery. Present day pain resulting from the original injury would be treated in a similar way to a slipped disc.

Sciatica

Sciatica is one of the most prevalent forms of back pain and is caused by undue pressure on the sciatic nerve. The nerve starts at the spinal cord in the lower back and divides to run down both legs. The commonest reason is pressure from a slipped disc in the lumbar area of the spine. Often the pain is felt suddenly and very acutely after the person has jerked awkwardly or moved a heavy object, but it may start more gradually, perhaps because of changes in postural habits. (See also Back pain and slipped disc pages 51–52, and Lumbago page 65, where various treatments are discussed).

Shingles and postherpetic neuralgia

Shingles is a common example of neuralgia where the nerve pathway becomes inflamed due to an infection. Deep pain is felt along the site of the rash in the acute stage and the pain is always one-sided. In about 20 per cent of those infected, the pain continues well after the other symptoms have disappeared. This complication, called 'postherpetic neuralgia' (PHN), causes severe nerve pain often described as a burning, throbbing and shooting sensation. PHN is diagnosed if the pain persists, or returns, within three months of the original rash. The area remains very tender when even the lightest touch from clothing or a slight breeze causes agonising pain. This extreme sensitivity is known as 'allodynia' and may be accompanied by intense itching. The risk of developing PHN increase with age and it is probable that about 50 per cent of people over the age of 60 years will continue to feel chronic discomfort. PHN cannot be cured, but the earlier it is treated, the more likely it is to improve. Most people experience improvement over time, depending on the duration of the pain. If a person is suffering from PHN six months after a shingles infection, then there is a 60 per cent chance of improvement over the following year. If pain has lasted for more than a year, only a few sufferers will experience an improvement, and if pain is still being experienced after three years, it is very unlikely indeed that the sufferer will ever be completely free from PHN pain.

Sickle cell disease

This genetic condition is found almost exclusively in black people. It is a type of anaemia affecting the red blood cells, and is so-called because the cells appear sickle-shaped when examined under a microscope. The problem lies in the abnormal development of haemoglobin, the oxygen carrying part of the blood cell. Any activity or illness that reduces the level of oxygen in the blood, such as strenuous exertion or a respiratory infection, causes the haemoglobin to change. This subsequently leads to the characteristic alteration in the cell shape. The sickle-shaped cells are more fragile than normal-shaped cells and are destroyed by the body's immune system, giving rise to anaemia.

The disorder starts in childhood and affects both sexes equally. The symptoms show as yellow discolouration of the skin and eyeballs, fever develops, there is general weakness and breathlessness associated with anaemia, which causes great difficulty and discomfort when breathing speeds up during physical effort, and blood clots may appear anywhere in the body. The illness is chronic and cannot be cured. The person should always try to avoid exacerbating the problem because this can lead to a very distressing 'crisis' point in the disease, often needing hospital treatment and regular blood transfusions. (See page 209 for useful addresses.)

Slipped disc

(See Back pain, page 51.)

Spondylosis

This is the term given to the degeneration of joints and discs in the spine. The condition causes pain and restricted movement in whichever part of the back is affected, commonly the neck and lower back regions, where the joints may have become unstable. (See also Osteoarthritis page 47 and Back pain page 51.)

Stroke

A stroke is the common name for the illness that occurs when the blood supply to an area of the brain is interrupted (cerebral ischaemia, see page 64). The medical term for a stoke is cerebral-vascular accident or CVA. A stroke causes loss of body functions which may be sudden, transient or temporary, or permanent depending on the nature of the CVA. There are several types. For example, a major stroke causes severe loss of function which gets better slowly and often only partially, whereas a mild stroke causes less serious loss of function which improves quickly and leaves few residual problems. A transient ischaemic attack (TIA) causes mild loss of function that disappears quickly (within 24 hours) but may recur. TIAs can be the forerunner to a full stroke. The risk of having a stroke is increasingly common in older people, and uncommon before the age of 50 years.

The flow of blood in veins and arteries can be interrupted in several ways:

- when a blood vessel ruptures and bleeds into the surrounding tissue of the brain (haemorrhage);

- when a sudden, total blockage occurs in an artery caused by a floating blood clot (embolism) that has formed elsewhere in the system;

- when the blood supply is gradually impeded due to narrowing, furred up smaller arteries;

- or when clotting occurs directly in the blood vessels of the brain (thrombosis) causing a partial or total obstruction.

The immediate signs include:

- sudden loss of consciousness;

- weakness or loss of movement, usually on one side of the body only (hemiplegia) affecting one or more limbs, eyelids or mouth;

- confusion and/or loss of memory;

- loss of sensation in an area of the body such as the fingers;

- speech problems resulting in slurred or loss of words (dysphasia);

- swallowing difficulty;

- blurring or double vision and severe headache with possible nausea and vomiting.

The longer-term effects depend largely on how many brain cells have died; unfortunately, some symptoms may remain permanently giving rise to discomfort and painful joint movement. Home treatment is similar to that for a condition such as frozen shoulder (see page 59). A small number of people (about 5 per cent) develop central post-stroke pain (CPSP), usually several months later. CPSP is a nerve pain, which feels like a burning or throbbing sensation, often brought on by touching the affected area particularly by a cold object. Strong painkilling drugs seem to have little effect, but treatment with anti-depressant tablets can make a real contribution as this group of drugs work better at combating nerve pain. Doctors recommend that treatment is started at an early stage as this improves the chances of easing this type of pain. Do not delay in the hope that it will go away with time because this is unlikely.

Syringomyelia

Syringomyelia is a rare disorder affecting the central part of the spinal cord, included here more as a contrasting illustration of a disease where people *lose* their sense of pain. Irregular cavities are found in the spinal cord of people with this disorder, together with excessive amounts of connective tissue. The cavities affect the nerve paths in the cord producing the characteristic, pain-loss symptom in the limbs, including heat and cold; however the merest sense of *touch* is retained. In addition, there may be a degree of muscle wasting in the limbs. The lack of sensitivity to painful experiences often leads to accidental wounding and burning. The disease is slowly progressive, so the best way people can help themselves is to be aware of their own vulnerability and to take responsibility for maintaining their own general health.

Tendinitis

Tendinitis means inflammation of a tendon, the fibrous end to a muscle where it is attached to bone. The sheath area surrounding the tendon is usually implicated also (tenosynovitis).

Trigeminal neuralgia

(See Neuralgia, page 69)

Ulcer

An ulcer is an inflamed opening in the surface skin or mucous membrane lining of internal cavities, such as the digestive (alimentary) tract. The two types share common characteristics:

- damage must have occurred at the site;
- immediate healing is delayed and thereafter the area does not heal easily;
- the floor of the ulcer is depressed (before healing starts) due to loss of tissue;
- there is a defined edge where the healthy tissue ends.

Any significant illness or general debility that lowers the healing function is likely to increase the possibility of an ulcer forming; for example, the ageing process, poor circulation, diabetes, gout. In addition, ulcers at specific sites may have other contributing factors, described below.

At first an ulcer looks yellowish at its centre but as it starts to heal the floor develops a form of granulation tissue. This healing tissue is composed of masses of new cells and the healing core appears to be brighter red in colour due to increased capillary blood vessels. In contrast, the new growth of skin cells makes the edge look bluer in colour; the line of new skin gradually moves inwards. The granulation tissue is more fibrous in texture than normal body tissue and as the edges draw together a raised, puckered appearance may result (proud flesh).

The sites and seriousness of ulcers vary; for example, the alimentary tract ulcers occur throughout the digestive canal, but the types may have different causes.

Mouth ulcers

Almost everyone has experienced ulcers in the mouth. These can develop on the inner lips or cheeks, the tongue or roof of the mouth. Sometimes they appear following an accidental bite or burn which seems to heal less well if the person is feeling 'below par'. They are also associated with stress, a deficiency in folic acid and vitamin B_{12} and chronic bowel disease. In the acute stage mouth ulcers are very painful and may recur regularly; however, their presence is rarely serious and their unpleasant effects can be treated with over-the-counter gels designed to anaesthetise the area and promote healing. Multiple ulcers and erosion, particularly at the corners of the mouth, are called stomatitis.

Stomach ulcer

A stomach (or gastric) ulcer is quite common and if untreated can be a serious illness. Data from autopsy records show that about one person in 20 has had a stomach ulcer at some time in their life. It is most likely to form near the opening to the small bowel (pyloric orifice) because it is here that digesting food causes the most friction. A complete picture relating to the causes is not fully understood; however, some influencing factors are known and it is probable that several of the following criteria are involved in triggering an ulcer:

- the condition is more common in men than women;

- the number of people affected increases with age;

- many affected people smoke or drink alcohol in excess, have increased levels of stress and eat irregularly;

- some alteration has occurred in the formation of mucus;

- bile juices might reflux backwards from the duodenum section of the bowel immediately below the stomach valve, damaging the gastric wall lining;

- a bacterium *(Helicobacter pylori)* may be present;

- there could be reduced blood flow supplying the mucosal stomach lining;

- damage might occur in the mechanism (linked to prostaglandin production) that helps to protect the mucosal cells.

This latter factor also increases the risk for people who take non-steroid anti-inflammatory drugs (NSAIDs) because the drugs contain prostaglandins, as does the long term use of other drugs such as aspirin (which irritates the lining of the stomach). Gastric ulcers tend to be small in surface size but can be deep as they eat into the mucosal lining, and eventually the muscular wall, of the stomach. Minor ulceration may heal with few symptoms. A larger, chronic ulcer causes a range of symptoms:

- gnawing pain in the upper abdomen, which is more likely to be felt when the stomach is empty (due to acid burn);

- nausea, which may develop after food is eaten;

- stale blood may be passed showing as tar-like stools;
- vomit may be streaked with fresh blood or show a dark sediment like coffee grains.

An emergency situation could arise if the ulcer invades a blood vessel causing blood to haemorrhage into the stomach. Or peritonitis (inflammation of the abdominal cavity) may develop if the ulcer perforates the stomach wall allowing acid to flow into the cavity. Another complication can occur when, during natural healing, the muscles at the pyloric opening become constricted due to scarring (called pyloric stenosis). This results in a slower passage of food and eventual enlargement of the stomach.

Symptoms from a stomach ulcer sometimes mimic a stomach cancer, especially if it seems slow to heal. Treatment focuses on an appropriate diet – for example, cutting out spicy foods and eating regular meals, using antacid medication, ceasing to drink alcohol, stopping smoking any form of tobacco, reviewing lifestyle and identifying emotional and stress-inducing triggers. It is also important that the possibility of the symptoms being caused by a malignant growth is ruled out. Full healing should take place over a few months, but the ulcer is likely to return if the habits that contributed to its formation continue. More severe cases may require surgery.

Duodenal ulcer
Ulcers form in the area where the stomach joins the small intestine (the duodenum) because the gastric juices here are at their most acidic. The chances of developing an ulcer in these first few inches is three or four times more likely in men than in women. In addition, studies have found that people with duodenal and stomach ulcers are most likely to have the blood group O, and there is often a family connection. The symptoms are also similar in the two types, with the pain from a duodenal ulcer most obvious below the ribs and in the early hours of the morning. It tends to start a few hours after a meal and remains until more food is eaten or an antacid medication is taken. The presence of food (or the medicine) dilutes the effects of the strong acids produced by the lower end of the stomach and the duodenum walls. The ulcer may niggle away for weeks and then symptoms subside; however, it usually recurs unless properly treated. The causes, treatments and complications are similar to those of a gastric ulcer. An additional complication may arise if the

ulcer penetrates the back wall of the duodenum into the pancreas causing inflammation (pancreatitis) and severe back pain.

Varicose ulcers

Most commonly found in older people, the ulcer appears in the lower
legs and is a complication of chronic problems with varicose veins. The
surface skin breaks down leaving a weeping sore which, although not
very painful in itself, can become infected, causing a great deal of discomfort. Varicose ulcers happen primarily because the surface skin has
become fragile and eczema-like due to poor circulation, it is then easily
broken following an accidental knock or scratch (sometimes from fingernails to relieve itching). Treatment involves resting the limb in a raised
position. Hygienic care is important when dressing the sore. In the long
term, if the ulcer is slow to heal, a skin graft may be necessary.

Other types of ulcer

Other less common types of ulcer may arise in different parts of the
body. They can be caused by illnesses such as tuberculosis, syphilis,
typhoid-like bowel diseases, as a complication of a malignant tumour, as
a result of a weakened nerve (trophic ulcers) and pressure sores (decu-
bitus ulcers) in immobile patients. Each type would be treated in accord-
ance with its cause.

Whiplash

A whiplash injury occurs when the neck is jerked violently forwards then
backwards (the term describes the action of a cracking whip). The most
common cause is when a person, sitting in a stationary car, is thrown
about because their car is struck from behind by another vehicle – usually unexpectedly – giving them no chance to brace themselves for
the impact. The resulting damage is liable to affect several areas in the
neck: the bones of the vertebrae may be crunched, the discs separating
the bones may be dislocated, and/or the neighbouring nerves may be
crushed.

Symptoms of whiplash include headaches, pain and rigidity in the neck,
pins and needles, numbness and weakness in the arms and hands,
along with a general feeling of being anxious and unwell. The symptoms
may be present immediately after the trauma, or they may be noticed a
while after the event. Treatment would include drugs to reduce the pain

and inflammation, physiotherapy and a collar to support the neck and restrict movement.

Wryneck

This is a disorder in which the head is twisted to one side. This is often as a result of a previous injury such as a healed burn scar, or paralysis of the neck muscles, or a spasmodic contraction of neck muscles (like cramp) or torticollis (a shortness of the sternomastoid muscle joining the breast and collar bones). The main form of treatment is by physiotherapy, or surgery where appropriate to ease the scarring.

Conclusion

This chapter has introduced you to some of the many disorders and illnesses that cause pain. It may have felt a bit like reading a medical dictionary in its descriptive style and some of the detail has been technical, but knowing more about the reason for pain should help you to understand better why you feel discomfort. The next chapter looks at how pain is assessed and diagnosed.

For more information

- Specific disorders: where there is a reference to 'useful addresses' above, details of one or more specialist organisations can be found in the alphabetical list starting on page 201.

- General support: several organisations (see address list) offer help and advice to sufferers and health care professionals, such as:

    △ The Pain Relief Foundation, offers a wide range of information leaflets covering, for example:
    ▲ Cancer pain
    ▲ Dental pain
    ▲ Diabetes pain
    ▲ Electrical stimulators
    ▲ Facial pain
    ▲ Low back pain
    ▲ Migraine
    ▲ Phantom limb pain
    ▲ Shingles and post herpetic neuralgia

▲ Pain following stroke
▲ Trigeminal neuralgia
△ Action on Pain
△ Pain Support
△ The British Pain Society.

• *Caring for someone with cancer,* by Toni Battison (2002). Age Concern Books.

• Support groups: several national organisations can help put people in touch with charities and benevolent funds:

    △ The Patients Association (address see page 208) keeps a database giving contact details and background information on over 1,000 self-help and patient organisations throughout the UK. Access their website at www.patients-association.com by keying in relevant details to describe the type of organisation you are seeking. In addition to the database, The Patients Association website carries a wide range of other patient-related information.
    △ The Association of Charity Officers (address on page 202).
    △ Charity Search (address on page 203).

3 Diagnosis and assessment

Earlier chapters covered how the body responds to pain, introduced you to the various types of pain and described many of the common causes. This chapter moves forward to look at some of the reasons why people react to pain differently, and explains how your pain is likely to be assessed. Over the years you may have heard people use an assortment of words to describe your discomfort: volume, intensity and pain levels are common examples, and, although the terms may have subtly different meanings, they all serve a similar purpose – to help professional people find out how badly you are hurting, to evaluate the effectiveness of a treatment or to explain as clearly as possible some of the anomalies arising from your pain.

Reaction to pain

People react to pain very differently and a number of physical and psychosocial issues play a part. The following examples offer some explanations, however, it would be very difficult to pinpoint every circumstance that might influence behaviour.

- **Cultural values** Cultural background can profoundly influence how we express our pain. People in many societies are expected to hide their discomfort and to show no hint of pain. In the UK, past generations were very intolerant of 'cowardice', particularly during a crisis. Even in modern times children are still encouraged to 'be brave', and adults told to 'show a stiff upper lip'. However, not all cultures follow this view – for example, some peoples are expected to verbally express their discomfort and pain is often accompanied by moaning and crying.

- **Emotional sensitivity** Inner feelings can make a huge difference to how a person deals with their pain. 'Self-talk' plays a part here. A person who feels mentally 'strong' is automatically sending messages to the pain centre in the brain that they are 'in control' and 'coping well'. On the other hand, someone who is feeling emotionally fragile is likely to be transmitting the opposite senti- ment, subconsciously persuading themselves that they are not managing well. For example, if your mood is buoyant you are far less likely to develop a tension headache.

- **Previous pain history** A person's attitude towards pain is influ- enced significantly by how well their pain was dealt with in the past. Good pain control helps people build an armoury of coping skills. But negative past experiences can make you believe that pain is a thing to be feared. For example, a painful childhood visit to a dental surgery is likely to leave very unpleasant memories.

- **New or recurrent pain** The type of pain, whether acute or chronic, can have a bearing on how swiftly a person takes action. New and unexplained pain, providing it causes sufficient distress, is unlikely to be ignored. In contrast, the return of a chronic pain may merely register as a nuisance and receive lower priority, however bad it feels.

- **The gravity of the cause** If a serious illness has already been diagnosed, such as a malignant tumour, concern about the prog- nosis usually dictates how urgently a person reacts: in the majority of cases people are likely to seek immediate help if only because they wish for reassurance.

- **Attitude to life** A person who believes in taking positive steps to direct their life tends to take action more quickly than someone with a negative, fatalistic attitude, who may delay seeking help.

- **The time of day** Certain disorders are known to be more 'active' at particular points in the 24-hour cycle. This phenomenon may increase a person's anxiety and susceptibility to feeling their pain. The early hours of the morning, in particular, seem to be the worst time for discomfort perhaps making pain, which was bearable during the day, seem less tolerable at night. There are physical and psychological reasons for this, in most cases. For example, gastric acid is more concentrated at night when there is less fluid to dilute it so the pain of a duodenal ulcer is more active. There is also less input to the brain (in the quiet of the night) which allows pain impulses to dominate without the negating effects of sur- rounding activity and distraction.

Pain response is a complex and unique business. No two people will behave identically and even the same person might show variable responses on different days. The illustrations above are just some examples of the many factors that can influence a person's approach and reaction to pain. Several studies over the years, questioning patients receiving surgery, have reported a number of situations where pain appears more difficult to regulate; for example, when the person:

- is very frightened;

- has lost trust in the benefits of the treatment;

- feels out of control;

- or is unsure about what is happening to them.

Conversely, it has been shown that if people are given clear explanations about how they will be treated, they are more likely to respond positively. As long ago as 1964 a study by Egbert and colleagues, found that 'a pre-operative discussion of probable post-surgical treatment and possible pain halved the requirement for morphine and reduced the time to discharge'. Many subsequent pieces of research into patient care have confirmed this understanding.

One of most important aspects in pain control is the overriding effect the brain can exert throughout the whole system. Gate Control Theory explained the role it plays in controlling the effect, because emotional pressures (anxiety and fear) help to keep the 'gateway' open, while cognitive thoughts and calming actions encourage it to close, reducing the pain. The brain is also able at certain times to trigger the release of chemicals in the spinal cord. These substances, called neurotransmitters (noradrenaline and serotonin) transmit messages between nerve cells and it seems that an increase in the level of these chemicals helps to damp down pain. This device, along with other forms of chemical action mentioned in Chapter One, increases or modulates sensitivity to pain. These mechanisms have been likened to turning up or lowering the volume control in a sound system, and they play an essential role in our self-protection co-ordination: the higher the volume the quicker the body takes action.

The effect other barriers to pain management can play is covered more fully later in this chapter.

Pain thresholds

One of the anomalies that surround pain perception is why one person appears to feel pain less strongly than another in similar circumstances. No single reason has so far been identified; it is thought that pain perception is more likely to stem from a combination of factors. These may include:

- **The state of an individual person's nervous system** This can be accounted for by at least two factors – genetic make-up and degenerative consequences. Some people's nervous system is naturally more efficient than other people's. Over the years, however, everyone's essential nerves lose some of their power to conduct stimuli. Our brains also become less efficient at processing pain, but the rate of progression varies in individual people. In addition, it is recognised that nerves are 'blood thirsty' organs requiring a constant and plentiful supply of blood, which may be reduced in older people with furred up arteries.

- **The consequences of reducing health** Younger, healthy people are usually better able to deal with trivial injuries than the majority of older people, who tend to become less robust. In addition to the general effects of ageing, some people become weakened further by chronic, disabling illnesses.

- **Personality** Where people are of similar age and comparable health, inherited personality may be a motivating factor. People with stronger willpower – the so-called Type A personality – often try harder to conceal what they perceive as deficiencies in their make-up; whereas Type B people tend to be more sensitive and less likely to disguise their feelings. It is believed that people who can *tolerate* pain better, probably *feel* less pain.

- **Mitigating circumstances** In extenuating conditions a person with a focused mind is often capable of blocking out all unpleasant stimuli. It has been observed that soldiers in battle have continued to fulfil their mission, despite severe injuries, because the over-riding struggle to win and their instinctive sense of survival masks all else.

Diagnosing pain

Fear of pain is an anxiety that is commonly shared, so anything beyond a mild and temporary ache will send most of us in search of medical attention. As you reach this chapter you may be long past the diagnostic stage of your illness and more accustomed to dealing with the consequences of pain. However, don't be tempted to skip over this section because reading the information about tests and investigations could help you learn more about the diagnostic process, especially if there were points about pain assessment that you did not fully understand. It isn't too late to ask questions about why certain tests were performed and to have the results explained again. The medical team will be very aware that in a time of great stress people find it difficult to focus clearly on what is taking place, and that you may well have attended the surgery or hospital appointments in a daze. It is important too not to underestimate the extent to which preoccupation with pain itself can affect your memory and ability to concentrate on other things.

Similarly, the range of treatment options often causes bewilderment. You probably know something about the different methods but may be less sure, for example, why certain therapies are recommended rather than an alternative choice; why treatments are used in combination; and why some work better with certain types of pain. (Treatment methods are covered in subsequent chapters.)

Early reporting

There are no grounds at all why any person need suffer pain unnecessarily, although there are many reasons why people do. For example, some people are unsure about how much pain should be borne before asking for help, or they believe that suffering pain is inevitable; another group may be fearful that their illness is worsening, or of enduring a further round of treatment; others hope that by ignoring the symptoms the pain may disappear spontaneously. None of these are wise sentiments to adopt. If you are experiencing any type of pain (whether new or recurrent) you are recommended to seek help at an early stage so the problem can be examined. Once the reason for the pain has been determined, the severity and its effects can be assessed, treatment commenced and future progress monitored for change. Medical intervention may not be able to eliminate the problem entirely, but all pain can be controlled.

One of the incentives for reporting pain promptly is that early reassurance often dispels undue anxiety. Not all pain is due to incurable diseases, or to your original condition. Other less dire causes may provide a simple answer and most are easily treatable. Neither does the amount of pain felt necessarily indicate that a disorder is getting worse. For example, tendon discomfort from an acute strain may be a quite separate entity from the chronic pain caused by arthritis, or a flare-up of inflammation can often be reduced quickly with a course of steroids.

Before you go for an appointment, think objectively about how you feel, and perhaps jot down a few notes. The clearer the information you can give to the nurse, doctor or therapist, the easier it will be for them to define the pain precisely and decide on treatment. You may feel more able to cope with the stress of an appointment if someone accompanies you, even if they merely sit outside and wait. You are likely to be asked many of the following questions:

- Where does it hurt?

- Is the pain new or a recurrence of an existing illness?

- Does the pain move around, or is it always in the same spot?

- Does it get worse or better at certain times of the day?

- How would you describe it, for example, as a dull ache, a sharp continuous pain, or an intermittent stabbing sensation?

- Does it resemble other pain you have felt in the past – for example, toothache, or a headache, or a pulled muscle, or like having a baby?

- How bad it is? Try rating it on a simple scale of one to five, or use one of the assessment tools described later in this chapter.

- Does it improve with self-help or can you ignore it by using distracting strategies, for example, resting or walking, warming or cooling the affected area, concentrating on something other than the pain?

- Does the pain interfere with your day-to-day activities, for example, sleeping, eating, or enjoying leisure time?

Tests and investigations

What happens and why?

An investigation usually starts with the doctor or therapist asking about your pain and about relevant personal and family history and/or aspects of lifestyle that may have a bearing on the diagnosis. At the same visit, the specialist (family doctor, hospital consultant or non-medical practitioner) will usually do a physical examination. All pertinent signs, symptoms and history help them to get an overall picture; specific tests are then done to confirm the diagnosis and extent of the illness. The particular tests that are subsequently performed will depend entirely on the details given by you and what the doctor has observed – tests are never done unnecessarily. Some investigations can be done at smaller, community hospitals. For specialist diagnostic facilities, however, you may need to go to a larger hospital.

Blood tests

There are a number of blood tests used to help in the detection of many illnesses. None can give an outright diagnosis, only a pointer that something is not working properly. For example, a sample of blood can provide a visible picture of blood cells in the case of suspected leukaemia or sickle cell anaemia. Collecting a blood sample is considered a fairly routine procedure at the start of many investigations, and blood from the sample will be used to obtain several pieces of relevant information:

- **Full blood count** The number of cells (red, white and platelets) present in blood can indicate several facts. Red cells show haemoglobin levels and tell whether a person is anaemic; white cell count gives an indication of the state of the body's immune system and whether it is trying to fight an infection; and the platelets are checked because they play a significant role in helping to prevent bruising and bleeding.

- **Electrolytes** The levels of certain salts in the blood (in particular sodium and potassium) is critical. Checking these levels, called an electrolyte estimation, is an important indicator that something may be wrong because an imbalance occurs quickly when the body is unwell.

- **Urea** This substance is the chief waste product discharged from the body, in urine. The levels are measured to estimate kidney function.

- **Liver function tests** The liver is responsible for converting broken-down foodstuffs into materials essential for other bodily actions. The examination and measurement of protein and certain enzymes indicate whether the liver is working correctly and efficiently.

- **Special blood tests** These are performed when certain types of cancer are suspected. The detection of cancers that form in the reproductive tissue (testes, prostate or ovaries) is one example.

Biopsy

The various types of cancer and other illnesses can be diagnosed by looking at suspicious cells under a microscope, so this can be one of the starting points for diagnosis. The word 'biopsy' literally means 'the removal and examination of tissue from the living body for diagnostic purposes' *(Black's Medical Dictionary)*. In a nutshell this is exactly what happens! A small piece of living tissue is taken from the tumour or diseased organ and sent to the laboratory for diagnosis. It is possible that the suspected tissue will be removed at the first visit to the hospital, but the decision about how and when to perform a biopsy will depend entirely on the site of the suspected problem, however urgent the need is for diagnostic action. A full examination of the sample taken in a biopsy often takes several days. The results will then be sent to your GP or consultant, who will explain the findings and make sure you understand what will happen next.

Fibreoptic endoscopy

This test may sound very technical but it is simply a description of 'what happens and how'. A fibreoptic endoscopy is an investigation that enables a specialist to look into a hollow body cavity using an instrument called an endoscope. The device is fitted with a source of cold light that passes down a bundle of quartz fibres, sometimes up to 20,000 fibres at a time. Despite the large numbers of fibres carried by the tube, it is very narrow and extremely flexible.

The use of this technique has radically changed the way that doctors can view parts of the body that were previously inaccessible without a minor operation. The endoscope is manipulated from the outside, so that the operator can see and do whatever is needed. The fingertip controls enable the surgeon to remove mucus or a small piece of tissue for biopsy and the image is passed back to the outside by reflected light. Usually the examination can be done easily with a mild sedative and local anaesthetic.

This technique is commonly used in the following investigations:

- an **arthroscopy** to explore a painful joint;

- a **bronchoscopy** to examine the airways leading to and directly into the lungs with the tube being passed through the nose;

- an **oesophagoscopy**, **gastroscopy** and **duodenoscopy** to examine a particular part of the elongated gastrointestinal tract, the tube leading to and into the stomach (and just beyond) from the mouth;

- a **colonoscopy** to check the upper part of the intestinal tract, above the rectum, from the anal end. The lower part of the bowel (the rectum) is generally examined by the doctor in two ways: manually, with an inserted finger, and visually using a smooth, rigid metal instrument. This latter check is called a **sigmoidoscopy**;

- a **cystoscopy** to examine the tubes leading from the bladder (urethra) and the bladder itself. A light general anaesthetic may be given to avoid undue discomfort.

X-rays

Most people are familiar with general X-ray procedures such as the basic process described immediately below. However, the technique is also used more widely to help diagnose more complex problems in most body areas as the tests are relatively straightforward to perform and very informative.

- **Basic X-ray** This basic technique is used regularly as part of a routine medical examination, for example, the investigation of a suspected bone fracture. Short rays capable of penetrating soft tissue, such as muscle and fat, are beamed onto a photographic plate, thus giving a picture of what lies under the surface skin.

Hard tissue (bone) stops the progress of the ray, and so the bone looks denser, and therefore stands out against the softer tissue making cracks easily visible.

* **Barium meal** This special X-ray involves swallowing a substance (often barium sulphate) that creates a contrast picture on the photographic film. If you are having a barium meal, you may be asked to fast overnight to ensure your digestive tract is relatively empty. Immediately before the X-ray procedure, you will be asked to swallow a cupful of barium and lie on a couch. You will then be linked to a TV monitor, and continuous X-ray pictures will be taken. The radiographer (the person trained to operate the X-ray machine) will move you into several positions to give a range of pictures from different angles. The X-ray film can then be developed and the frames separated for closer inspection. The test may not sound very pleasant, but it is not painful.

* **Barium enema** This special X-ray is identical to the barium meal, but taken from the reverse end of the digestive tract. The bowel must be completely empty so clear directions will be given beforehand about dietary control and the use of laxatives. The barium fluid, together with air, is inserted into the bowel via a tube and the X-ray pictures taken as required. The test can cause bloating and discomfort, and air will continue to escape after the test is completed.

* **Intravenous urogram (sometimes called a 'pyelogram' or IVP)** This test is designed to look at the kidneys and the tubes leading from the kidneys that carry urine down to the bladder (ureters). Under a local anaesthetic, a special (radio-opaque) dye, visible by X-ray, is injected into a vein. This dye can be photographed as it makes its way through the drainage system via the kidneys. The procedure gives a clear picture of the shape, position and structure of the kidneys and ureters, but it does have some disadvantages. It is quite a lengthy process and the dye may cause the patient's skin to look greenish in colour for a short while. There are certain risks connected with any procedure of this nature; for example, in exceptional cases there might be an adverse reaction to the dye being used. You should be given a full explanation by your doctor before agreeing to proceed. Do not hesitate to ask about any aspect of the test that is not made clear to you.

- **Cholecystogram** This test is similar to an IVP but is designed to check the function and shape of the liver, bile duct and gall bladder. The radio-opaque dye is usually given by mouth.

- **Arteriogram, venogram and lymphogram** These tests use radio-opaque dyes to examine arteries, veins and the lymph system.

- **Mammogram** This X-ray is best known for its preventive screening function rather than as a tool for diagnosis, but it may also be used in this way. The pictures are examined for signs of tumours or other abnormalities that show up before they can be felt.

Scans

Scanning is a relatively new procedure compared with the traditional X-rays and one that is much more exact. Scans were used mainly in the field of cancer medicine: as a means of diagnosis (or to rule out a suspected tumour) and, especially, to give a baseline picture of the size, position and shape of any tumour present so that subsequent scans could be taken to monitor the effects of treatment. Increasingly, scans are being used more widely as an investigative tool in other areas of medicine.

The scanning process uses a number of different techniques described below. Computed tomography (CT) and magnetic resonance imaging (MRI) scanning use a similar manoeuvre where the whole body, or a smaller section, is moved slowly through a tunnel-shaped cavity while 'pictures' are taken. Most modern machines require the patient to be very still (with breath held) for only a few seconds. Although the process does hold some fears for people who are concerned about being shut into a narrow space, in reality many people say afterwards that it was less frightening than they had imagined. The staff operating the equipment will be very supportive and are always present if help is needed. The different scanning processes include:

- **Computed tomography (CT)** This is a special X-ray technique that enables clearly focused images to be taken in a particular plane showing the structures present at that level. Thousands of readings are taken in wafer-thin slices, half to one centimetre apart, so that the resulting picture (a tomograph) can be viewed as a series of cross sections of the body. X-rays are beamed across the tunnel where the patient is lying and through their body to be picked up by special sensors. The information is fed into a computer that constructs a picture of what is present within each body slice photographed. The tomograph gives a very valuable image of internal organs, for example, showing how a tumour mass may be distorting an organ or where the lump is of a different density to the surrounding tissue. Occasionally, special X-ray-sensitive dyes and fluids are inserted or swallowed to intensify the image.

- **Magnetic resonance imaging (MRI)** This is another technique that uses computers combined with powerful energy waves to produce a picture of a body area. In this procedure radio waves (instead of X-rays) are intermittently beamed at the body within a strong magnetic field causing a certain alignment of body cells (atomic nuclei) in the direction of the field. The technique employs the knowledge that differing structures of tissues give off different vibratory energy signals. These signals are then built up by the computer to form a picture of the tissue being investigated in any body plane, similar to CT. MRI is very useful in neurological examinations, but is used less in cancer detection or continuing care. The process may take some time and can be very noisy. Great care must be taken to check beforehand whether patients have any metal in their body, such as pins repairing fractures, or pacemakers, because the strong magnetic pull exerted by the energy waves may damage their function.

- **Radioactive isotope scan (sometimes called nuclear medicine)** In this test, minute quantities of radioactive material called isotopes are used as diagnostic tools to detect abnormalities. The process works because many substances found naturally in the body, such as iodine, can be used to carry radioactive materials that emit radiation. The isotope, together with its carrier, is introduced into the body by an appropriate method, usually via a vein, and after a short while a special camera scans the radiation being given off. The distribution of radiation is then measured and recorded to give a visual plot indicating high and low spots. This technique can be used to detect rare kidney tumours in children and to view changes in bone tissue where secondary cancer may have formed. The technique requires specialist equipment so patients may have to travel to a dedicated centre for the test. Isotope testing is also used in other forms of diagnostic medicine as well as cancer detection, for example, to measure the action of the thyroid gland.

- **Ultrasound (ultrasonic) scans** This test is most commonly associated with pregnancy; however, it is also used as a way of examining many other organs. Ultrasound has several advantages: it is non-invasive, swift, inexpensive, versatile and, because it is harmless, it can be repeated as often as necessary. The technique is rapidly replacing other investigative processes such as radiography and isotope scanning. Ultrasound is so refined that very small lumps can be detected and the operator can carry out a needle biopsy using ultrasound as a guide. In particular, organs deep in the abdomen, the breasts and testicles can be checked by ultrasound technique with little discomfort. A water-soluble jelly is spread over the area to be examined to help the instrument make good contact with the skin. Sound waves that move at frequencies far above the level heard by the human ear (15 kilocycles per second) are bounced from a scanning head through the body tissue (via body fluids) and back to their source. The head of the instrument is moved steadily over the area and the picture is transmitted back to the analyser, which converts electronic signals into live pictures on a screen. The still pictures can be printed for future examination.

Assessing pain

The procedures and resource materials described in the following sections to illustrate pain assessment methods have (unless otherwise stated) been reproduced with kind permission of the Pain Clinic at Addenbrooke's Hospital, Cambridge. The staff team has selected these particular systems and charts because they suit a wide variety of patients' needs. You might find different versions and services at other pain clinics in the UK, but the end purpose will be the same. In addition to the pain clinics found at most larger hospitals, which are usually consultant led, a growing number of community-based pain clinics are springing up around the country. These clinics tend to deal with certain types of chronic pain, are often led by specially trained GPs and may be held at a surgery or health centre or a smaller, community hospital.

In the past, pain assessment was less formal than it has now become. Nurses and doctors observed patient behaviour, asked brief questions and generally relied on their own judgement to decide the level and type of pain that might be present. For various reasons they sometimes got it wrong. Consequently, patients often continued to suffer pain unnecessarily or were overdosed with needless analgesics. Either way the patients, perhaps out of fear or feelings of helplessness, rarely disputed the treatment they were given. Nowadays, proper pain assessment tools are used in most hospital settings, alongside the physiological signs and the important verbal information supplied by the patient. Hopefully, the likelihood of error and bias is now reduced.

The value of accurate pain assessment

The benefits of using a recognised and effective pain assessment procedure are many, for example:

- It provides a set of charts and questions which enable patients to communicate to staff using a consistent and standard format.

- It allows patients to feel in control.

- It gives a sense that pain management is a shared goal.

- It provides written evidence for future comparison.

- It allows all staff members to evaluate the efficacy (or failure) of their prescribed treatments against those of other team members.

- It helps people achieve a better quality of life.

- Any side effects can be documented and assessed.

However, it is not possible to use objective assessment tools successfully with patients who cannot communicate effectively; in particular, infants, people with dementia, people who are not conscious. For these groups, subjective methods, such as non-verbal assessment, are still employed.

Monitoring pain, for any category of patient, is not a foolproof practice because there are no methods that enable doctors to measure pain directly. All the tests currently used in diagnosis, such as blood or urine or neurological checks, provide clues to the reasons for the pain, but not its actual presence or intensity. Judgement by the patient is believed to be the most accurate report, but occasionally unco-operative patients do not give truthful responses. Various other barriers might also distort the process and must be taken into account when pain is assessed; for example, carers sometimes magnify – or minimise – the problem. (See also 'Barriers to successful pain management' page 113.)

Pain clinics

Access to specialist pain clinics is available through the NHS and private practice in many areas; however, as with numerous other categories of medical care, the extent of services offered for pain care does vary widely around the country. Initially, referral to a specialised centre is most likely to be via your general practitioner or a hospital consultant. A direct appointment with a private practitioner may be possible but it is probable that this independent consultant would also wish to liaise with your own doctor.

Not every person who complains of pain will be referred to a pain clinic as the majority of pain felt by older people can be successfully managed in primary care – especially if the person is well informed. The information below about pain clinics has been included to provide a rounded picture of the support that is available. If you are being treated by your GP, and you feel that more could be done, you may wish to use information taken from this book to help you discuss how your pain might be managed more effectively.

The main role of a pain clinic is to 'manage and control' your pain, whatever its cause. The treatment regime will aim to alleviate symptoms and work towards rehabilitation, to as high a degree as possible. However, no professional person at a pain clinic can ever promise full relief from pain or guarantee that it will not return. Achieving a better quality of life may be a more realistic aim and objectives might include a reduction in your medication and an increase in your use of self-help strategies which will enable you to live with the pain. Eradication of pain is not always a realistic goal, neither is finding a cause for your pain. Sometimes people have spent fruitless years moving from one hopeful investigation to another. Improving quality of life is often the last option, but even small changes in this area can be very positive.

In a statistical sense 'success rate' figures from pain clinics may appear to be low (maybe around 30 per cent of people treated). But in a broader sense, for many people, even a moderate reduction in pain is a bonus. You are also likely to be warned that when you have had pain for a long time it may take some while for it to subside. Treatment at a pain clinic usually takes many months and you may encounter quite long waits for both the initial and subsequent appointments.

Standard pain clinic procedure

The day-to-day arrangement at different pain clinics is likely to vary around the country, but new patients can expect to go through a procedure similar to that described here. The majority of clinics take a holistic approach, as it is generally believed that pain is inextricably linked in a bio/psycho/social relationship. In simpler words, pain cannot exist in isolation at a physical level alone – apart from the fundamental, biological process other emotional and social factors are invariably present (see Chapter One).

A typical routine, based on the practice at Addenbrooke's Hospital, includes:

• **Personal details** These are checked by a clinic receptionist.

• **Questionnaires** Forms are completed at each visit, asking patients about the effects of their pain (see below). Help is available if patients are unsure (or unable) to manage alone.

• **Assessment** A full assessment is usually done by a nurse called a Clinical Nurse Specialist (CNS), who is specifically trained and experienced in pain management. The CNS will start by asking a series of specific questions about the pain and its history and about any medication that the person is currently taking, or has previously taken. Patients may or may not be seen by a doctor on the first visit. If they do not speak to a doctor in the first instance it does not mean they are receiving care that is inferior in quality.

• **Physical examination** This check has been likened to a physiotherapy assessment, rather than a medical examination (see page 103). Extra clinical tests are rarely carried out at pain clinics because all the necessary diagnostic investigations will have been completed beforehand. Usually, the cause of the pain has already been established before a person is referred to the clinic.

• **Pain management** A programme of care will be recommended which is designed to promote functional independence. It is likely to include a combination of treatments similar to those described more fully in subsequent chapters, for example, medication, nerve blocking and use of specialist equipment, such as TENS (transcutaneous electrical nerve stimulating) machines.

Patients attend a clinic for as long as they or the medical team feel it is necessary; there are no set rules about the number of visits a person may be offered.

People you may meet in the pain clinic

In addition to meeting the CNS and the clinical consultant, over the course of the treatment you are likely to meet other clinic nurses and one or more specialist team members. For example:

- **A physiotherapist** Physiotherapists provide a range of physical treatments, including massage, heat treatment and exercise routines and advice about achieving daily comfort.

- **A clinical psychologist** This profession specialises in the emotional effects of pain. The suggestion that they talk to a psychologist or psychotherapist fills many people with alarm and they are often concerned that other people will think they are 'going mad'. If you have felt this way, you can be reassured that this is far from the case. As the bio/psycho/social phenomenon implies, when a person is in pain emotional feelings are always involved. The opportunity to talk over these sensitive aspects with someone who understands brain activity should be welcomed. A psychologist will take care to explain fully why your pain might have made you feel anxious and mentally low.

- **An occupational therapist (OT)** Occupational therapists work towards restoring and maintaining levels of independence and reducing the impact of illness. If your pain levels are so high that your work, personal life and family relationships are being affected (the 'social' part of the trio) an OT will help you to regain some control and a measure of normality.

- **A pharmacist** Pharmacists are trained and skilled to prepare and dispense all forms of medication.

Pain assessment tools

The array of pain assessment tools found at clinics forms part of an assortment of methods used in management programmes. Although there are known barriers, when performed properly, pain measurement techniques show a remarkably efficient set of results. The most vital element in the whole procedure remains the information supplied directly by you, the patient; the tools are used to complement what you say.

The key facts that a clinic team would wish to gather about the pain, from a patient or their carer, include:

- how severe it is;
- whereabouts it is;
- how often it occurs;
- whether it occurs on a regular basis;
- whether it is constant or remitting;
- whether the level of the pain changes;
- how long it lasts;
- what sort of pain it is (burning, crushing, stabbing, etc.);
- whether there are any factors that make it worse;
- the extent to which it affects the person's quality of life;
- what emotions the pain provokes.

Pain levels

The *level* of discomfort felt by someone is one of the measures used to decide the type and quantity of treatment necessary to manage their pain. But trying to describe an exact 'level' of pain is a difficult concept to define accurately. The person in pain may over- or under-estimate its severity, and the person they are telling may misjudge the intensity. The descriptions given below are commonly found on pain charts, so the definitions are well recognised as baseline measurements by most professional people that you might consult. You can use them also as a self-help means to help describe your own pain or to judge how poorly a family member feels.

- No pain
- Mild pain
- Moderate pain
- Severe pain.

Physical examination

The extent of the assessment carried out for each individual patient will be determined by their case history. However, a routine physical examination (performed at various stages during assessment) will cover many of the following checks:

- observation;
- relevant functional test, such as squat or hop for knee pain;
- active and passive ranges of movement;
- muscle tests to assess length, strength and control;
- neurological tests to assess, for example, reflex action, sensory levels, and mobility of the nervous system (eg leg raises);
- palpation to identify exact painful and tender areas;
- accessory movements (movements of joints that cannot be performed by the patient themselves).

In-patient monitoring

Where patients are likely to experience pain, for example, because of forthcoming surgery, they are told about pain assessment methods at an early stage in their relationship with the hospital. A record of pain levels is kept throughout their stay in hospital, and the patient may be asked to continue monitoring at home for up to three months after being discharged. The same chart is used during this time to ensure continuity of care and language.

Visual chart

A laminated pain chart (**Figure 1**, page 104) is provided showing a dual, visual and verbal scoring system for patient use, with a third 'observer' scale for professional use only. Instructions telling patients how to measure their pain are printed on the reverse side of the chart (**Figure 2**, page 105). Note also the variation in shading, which provides an added visual indication from light to dark, as the pain level increases. The pictures indicating 'happy' to 'sad' facial expressions, again with colour coding, offer an important alternative method for patients who are unable to make use of the number/word prompts. A nurse checks each patient regularly and records the score for future reference. Where necessary, patients are helped to describe their feelings.

Figure 1 Laminated visual pain chart

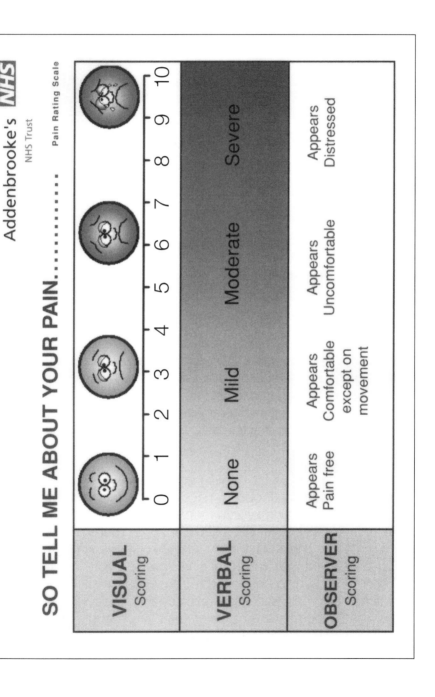

Figure 2 Laminated visual pain chart (reverse): instructions on how to measure pain

PATIENT INFORMATION

We need to measure your pain in order to provide you with the best treatment possible. There is a scoring system printed on the other side of this sheet.

This system will help you to tell us how much pain you are feeling now.

There are three scales printed overleaf:

     A series of faces

     A numerical scale; 0 to 10

     A series of descriptive phrases

You may use any of these or a combination of all three to best describe the level of pain you are feeling now.

You will be asked to repeat this at regular intervals and will be helped by a nurse who will record your score.

The observer scoring scale at the bottom of the page is for the use of nurses.

Most hospitals favour charts that are basic in style because they require minimal explanation. People who are in pain, or drowsy after an anaesthetic, also find it difficult to respond well to complicated assessment procedures.

Out-patient monitoring: Questionnaires

Patients who visit the Cambridge Pain Clinic are asked to complete three types of questionnaire during the course of their treatment.

Brief Pain Inventory (BPI) – new patients

The first BPI (**Figure 3**, page 107) asks patients to rate how their pain affects them over a time period, and in a range of situations where it is most likely to interfere with their lifestyle; for example, when walking, or sleeping, or working. In this format, patients gauge their *initial* pain levels as a benchmark against which future assessments can be measured. The chart uses a basic numerical system (from 1-10), with 10 being the severest level of pain they can imagine. There is also a visual, shaded bar, designed to help people identify the correct point on the scale, where using numbers may not be the best option.

Brief Pain Inventory (BPI) – follow up

The second BPI (**Figure 4**, page 108) is used at subsequent visits to the clinic, to monitor progress. This chart assesses any pain relief in evidence since the previous appointment, most likely to have been achieved by the treatments prescribed at the clinic. It asks patients to score their improvement (or otherwise) as a percentage of the relief felt. Again, a shaded bar is available for help those patients who need a visual aid).

Figure 3 PACS/BPI Assessment Form (page 107)

Figure 4 PACS/BPI Follow-up Form (page 108)

(Both reproduced with permission of Addenbrooke's NHS Trust and Pharmacia)

PACS/BPI ASSESSMENT FORM	BRIEF PAIN INVENTORY **NEW PATIENT** *Please circle your response or ask for help if you are having problems*
Hospital _____	1 Please rate your pain by circling the one number that best describes your pain at its WORST during the past week. 1 2 3 4 5 6 7 8 9 10 NO PAIN PAIN AS BAD AS YOU CAN IMAGINE
Date _____	2 Please rate your pain by circling the one number that best describes your pain at its LEAST during the past week. 1 2 3 4 5 6 7 8 9 10 NO PAIN PAIN AS BAD AS YOU CAN IMAGINE
Registration number _____	3 Please rate your pain by circling the one number that best describes your pain ON AVERAGE. 1 2 3 4 5 6 7 8 9 10 NO PAIN PAIN AS BAD AS YOU CAN IMAGINE
Patient's name _____	4 Please rate your pain by circling the one number that tells how much pain you have RIGHT NOW. 1 2 3 4 5 6 7 8 9 10 NO PAIN PAIN AS BAD AS YOU CAN IMAGINE
Year of birth _____	5 Circle the one number that describes how, during the past week, PAIN HAS INTERFERED with your: A. General activity 1 2 3 4 5 6 7 8 9 10 NO PAIN PAIN AS BAD AS YOU CAN IMAGINE
Diagnosis 1. _____	B. Mood 1 2 3 4 5 6 7 8 9 10 NO PAIN PAIN AS BAD AS YOU CAN IMAGINE
2. _____	C. Walking ability 1 2 3 4 5 6 7 8 9 10 NO PAIN PAIN AS BAD AS YOU CAN IMAGINE
Duration of symptoms _____	D. Normal work (includes both outside the home and housework) 1 2 3 4 5 6 7 8 9 10 NO PAIN PAIN AS BAD AS YOU CAN IMAGINE
Treatment _____	E. Relationships with other people 1 2 3 4 5 6 7 8 9 10 NO PAIN PAIN AS BAD AS YOU CAN IMAGINE
Consultant _____	F. Sleep 1 2 3 4 5 6 7 8 9 10 NO PAIN PAIN AS BAD AS YOU CAN IMAGINE
Source: Pain Research Group, Department of Neurology, University of Wisconsin-Madison Used with permission. May be duplicated and used in clinical practice. This data is collected for assessment of your pain. In addition, the information is entered into a national database for audit and research. This is anonymous. If you do not wish it to be used, then please inform pain clinic staff. **PHARMACIA**	G. Enjoyment of life 1 2 3 4 5 6 7 8 9 10 NO PAIN PAIN AS BAD AS YOU CAN IMAGINE

Figure 3 PACS/BPI Assessment Form

Figure 4 PACS/BPI Follow-up Form

PACS/BPI ASSESSMENT FORM

Hospital
_____

Date _____

Registration number
_____

Patient's name
_____

Year of birth _____

Diagnosis
1. _____

2. _____

Duration of symptoms
_____

Treatment
_____

Consultant
_____

Source: Pain Research Group, Department of Neurology, University of Wisconsin-Madison

Used with permission. May be duplicated and used in clinical practice.

This data is collected for assessment of your pain. In addition, the information is entered into a national database for audit and research. This is anonymous. If you do not wish it to be used, then please inform pain clinic staff.

PHARMACIA

BRIEF PAIN INVENTORY **FOLLOW UP**
Please circle your response or ask for help if you are having problems

1 How much RELIEF have pain treatments or medications FROM THIS CLINIC provided? Please circle the one percentage that shows how much.
100% 90% 80% 70% 60% 50% 40% 30% 20% 10% 0%

COMPLETE RELIEF   NO RELIEF

2 Please rate your pain by circling the one number that best describes your pain at its WORST during the past week.
1 2 3 4 5 6 7 8 9 10

NO PAIN   PAIN AS BAD AS YOU CAN IMAGINE

3 Please rate your pain by circling the one number that best describes your pain at its LEAST during the past week.
1 2 3 4 5 6 7 8 9 10

NO PAIN   PAIN AS BAD AS YOU CAN IMAGINE

4 Please rate your pain by circling the one number that best describes your pain ON AVERAGE.
1 2 3 4 5 6 7 8 9 10

NO PAIN   PAIN AS BAD AS YOU CAN IMAGINE

5 Please rate your pain by circling the one number that tells how much pain you have RIGHT NOW.
1 2 3 4 5 6 7 8 9 10

NO PAIN   PAIN AS BAD AS YOU CAN IMAGINE

6 Circle the one number that describes how, during the past week, PAIN HAS INTERFERED with your:
A. General activity
1 2 3 4 5 6 7 8 9 10

NO PAIN   PAIN AS BAD AS YOU CAN IMAGINE

B. Mood
1 2 3 4 5 6 7 8 9 10

NO PAIN   PAIN AS BAD AS YOU CAN IMAGINE

C. Walking ability
1 2 3 4 5 6 7 8 9 10

NO PAIN   PAIN AS BAD AS YOU CAN IMAGINE

D. Normal work (includes both outside the home and housework)
1 2 3 4 5 6 7 8 9 10

NO PAIN   PAIN AS BAD AS YOU CAN IMAGINE

E. Relationships with other people
1 2 3 4 5 6 7 8 9 10

NO PAIN   PAIN AS BAD AS YOU CAN IMAGINE

F. Sleep
1 2 3 4 5 6 7 8 9 10

NO PAIN   PAIN AS BAD AS YOU CAN IMAGINE

G. Enjoyment of life
1 2 3 4 5 6 7 8 9 10

NO PAIN   PAIN AS BAD AS YOU CAN IMAGINE

Hospital Anxiety Depression (HAD)

This questionnaire (**Figure 5**, pages 110-111) is designed to help patients analyse their emotional feelings in relation to their pain. At each visit the patient answers a series of multi-choice questions, using a tick-box format similar to those found in magazines. They are advised to do this spontaneously rather than pondering too long over their feelings. The questionnaire is scored easily by a member of the clinic team who overlays a transparent scoring sheet on top of the answer sheet. The maximum (worst) result that a patient could score is 21 points; the normal score acceptable to the clinic is 8-10 points. Any person scoring 10 points or above would trigger concern and clinic staff would expect to see a downward trend over the course of the treatment.

The methods shown in this section are examples only, favoured by the clinic in Cambridge. Hospitals in other areas no doubt use very similar tools. Readers may have come across different types including the following.

The McGill Pain Questionnaire (MPQ)

This particular model is widely used in both research studies and clinical practice. It utilises a large number of descriptive words, which patients are asked to rank using a numerical scoring system, arranged in four categories, covering the sensory, affective, evaluative and miscellaneous aspects of their pain. A shortened version is also available.

Visual body charts

This type provides front and rear drawings of the human body to enable patients to pinpoint the source of their pain. The body map is often accompanied by a tick-box style rating system, which may incorporate a number and/or word scale.

Analogue pain scales

These are simple, visual devices showing a continuum line about 10 centimetres long (**Figure 6**, page 112)). They can be used to indicate either pain relief or pain intensity. The starting point is given a label relating to a positive feeling, 'no pain at all' or 'least intensity', while the opposite point is labelled with words that imply the 'worst pain possible' or 'no relief'; some charts are marked with millimetre and centimetre spacing.

The **Figure 5** Hospital Anxiety Depression Scale (Reproduced with permission of Addenbrooke's NHS Trust and Pharmacia)

HAD Scale

Name: Date:

Doctors are aware that emotions play an important part in most illnesses. If your doctor knows about these feelings, he/she will be ale to help you more.

This questionnaire is designed to help your doctor to know how you feel. Read each item and place a firm tick in the box opposite the reply which comes closest to how you have been feeling in the past week.

Don't take too long over your replies: your immediate reaction to each item will probably be more accurate than a long thought-out response.

Tick only one box in each section

I feel tense or 'wound up':		**I feel as if I am slowed down:**	
Most of the time	☐■	Nearly all the time	■☐
All of the time	☐■	Very often	■☐
Time to time/occasionally	☐■	Sometimes	■☐
Not at all	☐■	Not at all	■☐

I still enjoy the things I used to enjoy:		**I get a sort of frightened feeling, like 'butterflies' in the stomach:**	
Definitely as much	■☐	Not at all	☐■
Not quite so much	■☐	Occasionally	☐■
Only a little	■☐	Quite often	☐■
Hardly at all	■☐	Very often	☐■

I get a sort of frightened feeling, as if something awful is about to happen:		**I have lost interest in my appearance:**	
Very definitely and quite badly	☐■	Definitely	■☐
Yes, but not too badly	☐■	I don't take as much care as I should	■☐
A little, but it doesn't worry me	☐■	I may not take quite as much care	■☐
Not at all	☐■	I take just as much care as ever	■☐

I can laugh and see the funny side of things:

As much as I always could ■☐

Not quite so much now ■☐

Definitely not so much now ■☐

Not at all ■☐

I feel restless as if I have to be on the move:

Very much indeed ☐■

Quite a lot ☐■

Not very much ☐■

Not at all ☐■

Worrying thoughts go through my mind:

A great deal of the time ☐■

A lot of the time ☐■

From time to time but not too often ☐■

Only occasionally ☐■

I look forward with enjoyment to things:

As much as I ever did ■☐

Rather less than I used to do ■☐

Definitely less than I used to ■☐

Hardly at all ■☐

I feel cheerful:

Not at all ■☐

Not often ■☐

Sometimes ■☐

Most of the time ■☐

I get sudden feelings of panic:

Very often indeed ☐■

Quite often ☐■

Not very often ☐■

Not at all ☐■

I can sit at ease and feel relaxed:

Definitely ☐■

Usually ☐■

Not often ☐■

Not at all ☐■

I can enjoy a good book or radio or TV programme:

Often ■☐

Sometimes ■☐

Not often ■☐

Very seldom ■☐

Do not write below this line

D (8 – 10) _____

A (8 – 10) _____

Figure 6 Analogue pain scales can be used to show pain relief or pain intensity

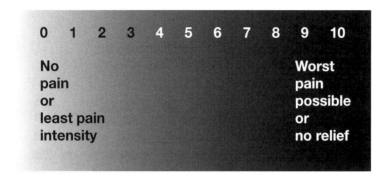

The patient is asked to point to the position which best describes their feeling, or in more sophisticated versions, to slide a cardboard indicator along. This basic type of tool is useful as a quick pain intensity guide because a precise number can be isolated and checked at regular intervals, but it does have limitations for use with patients who have difficulty concentrating and where a more comprehensive assessment is required. Pain relief scales sometimes work better than pain intensity scales because patients find it easier to define relief of pain than its intensity.

Pain diary

Recording the intensity and frequency of pain is possible using a 'pain diary', often designed as a booklet or specially marked sheet. Patients are asked to note several aspects of their pain, such as the level at regular intervals and where the pain is felt most severely, as agreed with their doctor, nurse, or therapist. The example on the facing page (**Figure 7**) could be used as a self-help tool. A word of caution, however: beware of letting a pain diary take over your life. The compulsion to fill it in every time you feel a twinge may distract you from focusing your energy on other more useful methods, and possibly slow down your progress.

Figure 7 A pain diary can be used to record a range of factors relating to pain

Date	Time	Site	Severity 1–10	Other symptoms	Emotional feelings	Activity at time

Leaflets

Most hospital departments offer a comprehensive range of patient information leaflets, produced internally by clinic staff, or by drug companies or from major pain-combating charities. For example, the Pain Clinic at Addenbrooke's Hospital offers patients a selection of information leaflets. The leaflets are only available to clinic patients; however, you could ask about similar titles at your doctor's surgery or health centre or contact a national organisation (see useful address list, pages 201 and 208).

Examples include:

- Welcome to the pain clinic – patient information.

- Tricyclics for pain/sleep – patient information (tricyclics are a family of antidepressant medicine, used very successfully in the treatment of nerve pain, see page 69).

Barriers to successful pain management

'Why is it still hurting?' is a question asked by many people when their pain continues to be troublesome or returns again after a period of relief. The answer is that there are many answers, and when pain won't go away or comes back the person should be re-assessed. The aim this time will be to find out what might be hindering effective pain management. In reality there are few physical reasons why pain cannot be controlled, especially when a thorough assessment has been undertaken.

The main barrier for certain groups of people stems from their inability to communicate – either totally or adequately. Obvious categories include very young children, people with dementia, people with a different cultural language and people with learning difficulties. Of course this does not mean that the problem belongs with them; in reality the challenge lies with professionals who need to develop accurate skills of assessment and tools that measure and reflect non-verbal responses.

Apart from these groups, however, professional people also find that some patients, even when encouraged to describe how bad their pain feels, seem unable to do so accurately. When the reason for their 'reluctance' is explored further, it is often found that the cause lies within the patient's control. There are several well-recognised emotional or psychological explanations why some people resist giving the full picture. For example:

- they have a low expectation of what pain management can achieve;

- they are fearful of becoming addicted to an analgesic substance;

- they think that an increase in pain means the illness is getting worse and may disguise or 'blank out' their worries by pretending there is no change;

- they dread the tests or treatments, such as injections or computed tomography (CT), more than the pain;

- they assume that the doctor or nurse knows best and will deal with their pain without the need for patient feedback;

- they crave attention and this 'need' may influence how they respond – for example, by saying the pain is more severe than it is they may be seeking the offer of further appointments or for a nurse to come to their bedside more frequently;

- they feel that to express pain is a sign of weakness, or a punishment, or leads to a loss of independence.

If, for any reason, you have found it difficult to describe your pain accurately do not feel nervous or despairing. You can speak to any professional person within the medical team about your concerns and ask how you can have your pain re-assessed.

Making a complaint

If you are not happy with the services you receive from any organisation (NHS or voluntary agencies) or an independent practitioner, you should try to resolve the situation as soon as possible by speaking to the person involved. This could be the senior person on duty, or charity manager or the therapist. If you are still not satisfied and wish to take the matter further, contact a customer relations department or equivalent (a voluntary organisation will have a management committee) or the appropriate national body in the case of an independent therapist, and ask for details of their complaints procedure. Most NHS Trusts now have a PALS (Patient Advice and Liaison Services) Manager who will be able to help you make a complaint (for details ask at your doctor's surgery or health centre). The PALS Manager will also be able to tell you about a new service supporting those making a formal complaint about health services – the Independent Complaints Advocacy Service (ICAS), which has replaced Community Health Councils in England. The situation in Scotland, Wales and Northern Ireland is different and up to date information can be found on the relevant websites (see pages 208–210).

For independent advice on how to deal with a complaints procedure, contact your local Citizens Advice Bureau. Alternatively, Age Concern runs an Advocacy Service for older people in many areas. Contact your local Age Concern for details; or contact Age Concern's head offices (see page 214) for local details.

Conclusion

Diagnosing and assessing pain is not a clear-cut science, unlike the more straightforward procedures that can be employed in detecting many illnesses. Pain is an imprecise entity, with qualities that are difficult to describe. Reactions and feelings vary and sometimes patients are reluctant to seek advice. However, despite all of these obstacles pain is manageable. Having read this chapter, if you now believe that your pain has not been adequately assessed, it is probably a good time to consider re-visiting you doctor for further help and advice. The next chapter covers pain management options using self-help and orthodox treatments.

4 Dealing with the pain
– orthodox and self-help treatments

Dealing with the pain can be approached in different ways, depending on the nature of the pain and the unique needs of the individual person. Self-help, complementary therapies and over-the-counter remedies all provide excellent means to relieve milder discomfort. It is reasonably easy to buy and use non-prescription medication, and most people get to know from experience which product cures their headache best. Severe pain, on the other hand, generally calls for medical intervention to achieve satisfac-tory control. A pain specialist has the expert knowledge, skills and experience needed to treat acute or chronic pain, particularly the latter, as it requires a sustained approach. In many cases the 'pain expert' is likely to be your GP. However, as you will read later in this chapter the current thinking about pain management is 'multi-modal' where you (and the professionals) should aim to take full advantage of a range of interventions which reflect the multi-dimensional nature of pain.

Being realistic

When planning a pain relief programme, it is important that everyone works towards defining and agreeing a reasonable goal. It is not always possible, in every illness, to achieve a complete absence from pain and, where this is the case, it would be pointless and distressing to antici-pate a totally pain-free outcome. For instance, a person with chronic arthritis might feasibly aim for a pain level that eliminates most creaks and aches, and allows them to lead a comfortable lifestyle. Someone prone to unpredictable and devastating migraine attacks might feel that the means to delay the worst stage, at least until they could get home, would be a realistic goal. Never being without a migraine-specific pain-killer, therefore, could be a major confidence booster.

Jed is a local radio presenter
'My migraines arrive with astonishing speed and as I work in the public eye I can't afford to let my concentration falter. So over the years I have got into the habit of always doing a spot-check of my pockets when I leave the house – comb, wallet, tablets ... it's second nature now and my wife no longer needs to remind me.'

Setting goals is equally important if you are practising self-help therapies. If you feel happy about the level of support that a certain product or professional person is providing, then there is no reason to seek alternatives elsewhere.

Why is it important to treat pain at an early stage?

You may feel that treating pain is such an obvious and routine procedure that the question of treating it at an early stage is unnecessary; however, it is worth reflecting briefly on why moderate to severe pain should never be ignored. From an ethical viewpoint it is against medical values to allow people to suffer, but the following reasons are equally important for patient welfare and good pain control:

- Acute pain can turn into a chronic pain if it is uncontrolled or poorly treated.

- Acute inflamed tissue can become septic, leading to a possible spread of infection elsewhere. If poison gets into the bloodstream (causing septicaemia) the bacteria could damage vital organs, such as the heart, liver and kidneys. Severe septicaemia can be fatal.

- A person in severe pain tends to lie very still which may cause other problems to develop; for example, failure to breathe deeply and cough properly might lead to a chest infection; holding one group of muscles motionless can put additional stress on neighbouring groups; and inactivity causes all muscles to weaken.

- Acute pain causes anxiety and distress.

- Chronic pain is commonly cited as a major factor in depression.

- The effect of one person's pain often has much wider social repercussions, impacting on family, friends and colleagues. For example, relationships suffer, parents become irritable with children and people in the workplace tend to be less productive.

Rachel lives near to her elderly parents
'My mother is very bad at recognising her own limits. She will potter around for ages, then end up in so much pain from her arthritic knees. I've learned to pre-empt her sometimes, but it's difficult because she doesn't like anyone else to take over in her kitchen no matter how tired she is. And of course if she overdoes it, the pain stops her sleeping and she is even worse the next day.'

Orthodox or self-help treatments – which routes to choose?

It would not be sensible to make a snap decision about which treatment method might be the better option for you. Effective pain management theory promotes a blend of physical, psychological and social strategies (the bio/psycho/social approach) to boost the chances of achieving successful results. Most professional people adopt a pragmatic attitude and aim for the best combination. In line with popular advertising slogans why not 'mix and match' or 'pick and mix' for optimum choice.

The various techniques described in this chapter all bring relief in some form. Whenever a treatment programme is being selected the following points should be taken into account:

• the type of pain you are experiencing;

• the speed at which pain control is required;

• the best method by which a particular drug or drug cocktail can be introduced into the body;

• the need to keep any side effects to a minimum;

• your attitude towards pain relief, especially if the programme is likely to be a long-term exercise.

If you are practising self-help therapies alongside orthodox care, be sure to tell the nurse or doctor familiar with your case about the full list of treatments you are using. It is important that the different methods complement each other and that any potential risk from overdosing on a mixture of prescribed and over-the-counter medicines is assessed.

The 'self-help' philosophy is very important for many people because taking some personal control over their illness is often the impetus needed to move forward. It is generally accepted that self-help therapy, practised sensibly within well-recognised and safe parameters, rarely does any harm. Research carried out at Coventry University reported that 'people who became involved in managing their own illness can experience an improvement in health and general welfare … feeling less fatigued, less depressed and less anxious about their (chronic) illness.' *(Newsletter of the Guild of Health Writers,* March 2004). However, assuming a practical role in one's own day-to-day health care does mean investing energy and enthusiasm into getting the right balance. As a basic minimum you will need to understand how body systems work, build up an emotional self-awareness and find the time to check out the large range of therapies continually being promoted.

Finding help, health advice and product detail is not difficult these days, as consumers are bombarded with information. Look out for articles published by the local and national press, check the listed programmes to be broadcast on radio and television and investigate the huge range of information available on various websites. If you do not have access to the Internet yourself, this is an area where a younger family member or friend would no doubt be keen to demonstrate their knowledge and skills! Alternatively, the majority of public libraries provide Internet points and someone would help you go online. This type of media material is mostly well researched and aimed at the general public.

Zeta's story

Zeta has a chronic abscess in her psoas muscle (the strong muscle which passes from the lumbar region, through the pelvis and groin to the inner side of the thigh bone). This muscle is used to help us sit up from a lying position and Zeta says that on a bad day she feels severe back pain and right leg pain. She is also tired and has pain especially at the site of the abscess. In addition she struggles to sleep and feels drained. Zeta has had the chronic abscess for a year and a half.

On a good day Zeta doesn't feel pain at the site of the abscess itself, but she is still tired and continues to feel pain along her right leg and also has a slight back pain (on the right side).

For Zeta, the three key words that spring to mind in relation to her illness are 'continuous', 'restricting' and 'unbearable'.

The pain has repercussions for her family and friends because it makes everyone feel depressed, especially as there is uncertainty about achieving a cure.

The treatments that have worked best for Zeta over the years have been a combination of medication and self help:

Prescribed by the general practitioner or hospital consultant
- *Surgical operation to drain the abscess*
- *Antibiotic drugs*
- *Painkilling drugs.*

Self help treatment
- *Warmth from a cosy hot-water bottle.*

Zeta has not been referred to a pain clinic.

If you are unsure about how much to expect from self-help medication and therapies, or fear that you might make matters worse, bear the following points in mind:

- Whatever you try out, if it doesn't seem to be working after a reasonable period of time, then stop.

- Try one thing at a time in order to avoid confusion.

- Don't set too high expectations, as this won't achieve your objective and your distress may make the situation worse.

- If the pain level gets worse or other side effects become apparent you should speak to your own doctor.

The treatment methods described in the following section are not exclusive to either a medically orthodox or a self-help policy. The various methods, unless stated, are suitable for both approaches. Apart from its purpose, one of the main factors affecting treatment choice is often linked to ease of access, as some treatments are available only via prescribed medical care.

Medication

Medication usually underpins most pain control programmes, at least initially, so this method will be covered first. After a while it may be possible to reduce or discontinue your drug therapy as the pain becomes better controlled, or because it disappears naturally, or other techniques take precedence. Some people feel despairing at the thought of having to take drugs for perhaps the remainder of their lives. Fortunately, circumstances change so your case will be reviewed regularly to take account of new methods that have been developed, improved treatments, and the continually expanding skills and knowledge of practitioners.

The information given here is intended only as a brief outline of the main drugs used to control pain, to help you understand why medication is so important and what effects it can have. It is essential that some drugs be taken regularly to prevent a condition worsening, at least for a period of time, while other types become necessary only when aggravating symptoms develop. The doctor who prescribes the treatment will advise you in more detail.

It can be confusing for a non-medical person when the words 'drug' and 'medicine' are used to describe any form of medication, but they mean the same thing. Although there seem to be many drugs in use to treat pain there are, in fact, only a few main groups, described below. This apparent abundance of drugs is because:

- any one drug may be available in several variations;

- the doctor may try several drugs to find the combination which gives the best results with the fewest side effects;

- different manufacturers make the same basic drug but market it using their own trade name and colour of tablet. Think of medicine like coffee on a supermarket shelf – the names and the packaging are different but the granules look the same!

Professional people will give you considerable support but ultimately you are responsible for organising your own, or your relative's, drug routine. If you are a carer, be aware of another person's mental state. If there is any chance that they might be confused about which drugs to take, or how many tablets, do not leave any form of medication out for them to take later. The correct dosage must be supervised. If you or a relative are able to take the drugs safely but have difficulty opening containers, ask a pharmacist for details of specially designed tablet boxes with separate compartments that you can load with an advance supply. If you are concerned about getting the timing and doses right because you are taking several drugs, it might help to write out a chart as a memory aid.

The following basic rules apply to any medication:

- Follow the instructions given on the label.

- Never stop using a prescribed drug without taking medical advice.

- Take the dose regularly, at the stated times, to achieve the intended result.

- Never take more than the prescribed dose – if the pain persists or becomes worse seek advice.

- Store all medicines in a secure, locked place away from children and any person who may not handle the drugs safely.

- Always tell a pharmacist (or remind a doctor if you have not had a recent consultation) about other medication being taken; interaction between drugs or taking an excess amount because tablets with different names may contain the same active drug, can be very dangerous.

- Check repeat prescriptions to make sure that the type and dosage are correct, as mistakes do occur.

Clare is a GP
'Don't be too worried if you feel a bit low after reducing the dose of strong painkillers; as you pick up the threads of your life again the depression should lift. If it persists, speak to your doctor.'

How do drugs get into the system?

There are three main ways that drugs enter the body. The most common route is through the mouth. However, some drugs work better by being injected into the bloodstream and occasionally they are best absorbed via the skin. Most pain-controlling drugs are taken orally in tablet or liquid form but other methods are used; for example, skin plasters, suppositories, injections, intravenous drips and automatic syringe drivers. The list of absorption methods described below is comprehensive, so it is unlikely that any one person would be prescribed the full range.

- **Anal absorption** Suppositories are inserted into the back passage for slow release. Morphine may be given this way.

- **Absorption from the mouth** There are two 'sites' commonly used: the 'sublingual' area, where the tablet or aerosol spray is directed under the tongue to be absorbed quickly into the bloodstream, without the need for liquid and used primarily to relieve the pain caused by an angina attack; or the 'buccal' area, where the tablet is placed between the upper lip and gum to give a much slower method of absorption (four to six hours).

- **Intramuscular injection** This is given deep into a muscle, usually the buttock or thigh. Drugs inserted deeply into muscular tissue are absorbed slowly.

- **Intravenous injection** The liquid drug is injected into a vein, rapidly by syringe or slowly by a drip feed. Chemotherapy drugs are usually given this way.

- **Implanted lines** Devices, such as Hickman or central lines, are designed to be left in place for a period of time. A length of plastic tubing is inserted under the skin and fed into a large vein in the chest. Pain-relieving and other drugs are injected through the protruding end.

- **Oral swallowing** This route is used for tablets, capsules or liquid, from mild analgesics to quick-acting opium-based syrups.

- **Self-adhesive patches** This method, giving a slow absorption of the drug, is sometimes used to relieve severe pain. Fentanyl, a strong painkiller used as an alternative to morphine, is given this way.

- **Spinal cord route** This technique is used to relieve severe pain. A small catheter is inserted into the spinal cord by an anaesthetist and attached to a reservoir of the drug. A top-up dose of the drug can be injected whenever it is required.

- **Subcutaneous injection** The drug is inserted just under the surface of the skin, using a standard, hypodermic syringe or a modified version called a syringe driver. Subcutaneous injections are given for three main reasons: because a substance, such as insulin, cannot be given orally as it would be destroyed prematurely in the stomach; because the person is unable to take a medicine by mouth; or because swift action is needed, for example, the strong painkilling effects of morphine.

Common pain relievers

The main drugs used in the relief of pain come from several sources; common examples, such as morphine and codeine, are derived from opium while aspirin is made from acetylsalicylic acid. There are many drug options open to the doctor, so drug types, quantities and combination can change according to need. Painkillers can cause drowsiness so care must be taken. It is important to read the instructions, as it may not be safe to drive or take alcoholic drinks.

Painkilling medication comes in varying strengths and some can be very potent when combined; for example, certain non-steroidal anti-inflammatory drugs (NSAIDs) when taken together may result in serious side effects. Never mix drug combinations unless you have first sought advice from a professional person trained to understand the range of appropriate drugs and the dosages. Someone from your medical team or a pharmacist would be ideal. Please note: the information below is given as examples only and must not be used as the basis for self-prescribing.

Mild pain

Many painkillers, such as paracetamol, aspirin and NSAIDs (ibuprofen is one example) are available as prescription drugs from the hospital or a GP, or over-the-counter from a pharmacy. Some drugs have other functions in addition to their pain-relieving properties; for example, ibuprofen (eg Nurofen, Brufen) and aspirin help to reduce inflammation, and aspirin also lowers fever.

Moderate pain

NSAIDs, either alone or combined with paracetamol, can be used safely. At other times painkillers such as codeine are often prescribed in combination form with paracetamol (for example, solpadol). Many drugs that have the same effect will be marketed under different trade names (see above). However, and here is an example that illustrates the complexity of drug prescribing, some codeine-based drugs are less effective than others and yet they are regularly prescribed. They cause constipation and patients are misled into thinking that because they contain codeine they are very strong. Most moderate analgesics are available without a prescription, but those bought over the counter contain lower doses of codeine or its equivalent.

Severe pain

Opioids, such as morphine and its derivatives, are given to control severe pain (and NSAIDs can be effective with these drugs). Opium-based drugs are obtainable by medical prescription only as they are subject to very tight, legal controls. The dose of morphine is carefully adjusted to ensure adequate pain relief and to minimise unwanted side effects. Morphine treatment usually commences with a preparation aimed at bringing swift relief; the dose can then be repeated every four hours (and more frequently if pain persists). A 'double' dose may be given at night to avoid unnecessary disturbance. Once a suitable dose level has been established the doctor is likely to prescribe a slow release version that acts over a period of 12-24 hours.

Other medication

In addition to painkillers other drugs may also be prescribed to reduce inflammation and swelling and relax tense muscles – all factors that can make the pain feel worse. The use of non-analgesic drugs is called 'adjuvant' therapy. Adjuvant means a substance or treatment administered with another to enhance the effect. The way in which these drugs act alongside standard painkilling medication is complex and, in some cases, the exact reason why they work is unknown. The most commonly used drug groups are listed here.

Anti-convulsant and sedative drugs

This group is prescribed to help reduce tension by relaxing the body and the mind. Their exact function is not fully understood, but it appears likely that the drugs calm down abnormal nerve action in a similar way to stabilising convulsions. In particular they are used to ease the shooting pains that occur when nerves are damaged, for example in trigeminal neuralgia.

Anti-depressant drugs (tricyclics)

This group is prescribed to diminish the amount of pain impulses that travel along the nerve pathways to the brain. They are thought to work by enhancing chemical neurotransmitter activity in the pain pathways, which in turn moderates the 'volume' of the pain. Patients who are concerned about being prescribed anti-depressant drugs must be reassured that preparations from this group, such as amitriptyline, imipramine or nortriptyline, can be used very effectively in the treatment of nerve pain and are given in lower doses than would be prescribed to treat depression. Nerve pain is difficult to relieve using conventional painkillers alone, so a combination is usually prescribed for short-term care. Chronic pain tends to cause disturbed sleep so tricyclic drugs are also beneficial in this respect.

Anti-spasmodic drugs

This group is prescribed to reduce the spastic-like spasms, known as 'colic', caused by gas that might occur after an abdominal operation. They work by relaxing the smooth muscle, which makes the intestine contract.

Chemotherapy (cytotoxic) drugs

This group has a very specific use in the treatment of cancer. The drugs have a powerful toxic action which destroys body cells for three main reasons:

- to reduce the size of the tumour at its primary site;

- to kill breakaway cancer cells before they spread to other organs;

- to destroy secondary growths that may have already become established elsewhere in the body.

Reducing the size and shape of a tumour helps to alleviate the pain caused by pressure on nearby organs and nerves. Chemotherapy drugs are given in doses that aim to maximise damage to the malignant cells but minimise harm to healthy tissue.

Non-steroidal anti-inflammatory drugs (NSAIDs)

This group is prescribed to reduce pain and help to increase mobility. They are particularly useful in treating acute pain that flares up in a chronic disorder, such as arthritis. NSAIDs should not be confused with true steroids. Although they have a similar action, the drug composition is different, with far fewer side effects. However, NSAIDs should be used with caution in older people as they are more likely to cause adverse gastrointestinal effects (ulceration) in this age group. If you are being prescribed this type of drug and you begin to get heartburn, indigestion or abdominal pain, you must go and see your GP.

Steroid drugs

Steroids are prescribed to reduce swelling and chronic pain, especially where the inflammation has increased suddenly. They are thought to work by reducing tissue fluid, which lessens pressure on nerves and internal organs. In addition, they act on the pain-producing chemicals found in injured tissue.

Skin creams

These usually contain 'capsaicin', a substance derived from chilli peppers. Creams are used most effectively where their action affects localised, sensory nerve terminals found under the skin surface.

Tranquillisers (benzodiazepines)

These drugs, for example diazepam (Valium), are muscle-relaxants, prescribed to relieve acute muscular spasm commonly associated with back pain or musculo-skeletal injuries. Their action is only appropriate for short-term use as dependency is a known to develop if they are taken for lengthy periods.

Using cannabis

Certain non-medical drugs, such as cannabis, are believed to have pain-relieving properties. In recent years, studies have been carried out to find out whether cannabis can help with pain relief in illnesses such as multiple sclerosis but, as yet, there is no conclusive evidence to suggest that cannabis is any more effective in controlling pain than other prescription drugs. However, there is evidence to suggest that cannabis may be effective as a relaxant in the treatment of conditions such as anxiety and depression.

Drugs that have medical benefits (but are also used as recreational drugs) are categorised as prescription-only drugs. This means that a doctor is able to prescribe them in certain situations. The Prescription Only Medicines (Human Use) Order (2002), which gives details of prescription-only drugs, can be bought from Her Majesty Stationery Office (HMSO).

Over-the-counter remedies

This term covers the huge variety of non-prescription drugs, nowadays readily available in high street shops, supermarkets and by mail order, including both conventional medication and herbal or homeopathic remedies. It is important to be aware that even apparently harmless 'natural' remedies can cause other medicines you may be taking to behave differently. Wherever possible, try to obtain advice before buying products straight from the shelf or by mail order. In particular it is important to ask about possible interactions with the other medication and treatment you are receiving. A pharmacist would be a good person to approach as they are trained to be aware of how drugs act together and whether any new treatments would be suitable.

Side effects

Analgesic medicines do cause side effects, for some people. Constipation is often a problem; however doctors are aware of this and frequently suggest that laxatives are taken at the same time. Morphine may cause nausea. Medication can be taken to help ease the feeling, which usually improves as the system adjusts. A dry mouth is a minor side effect of morphine that can be helped by drinking plenty of fluids, sucking sweets, pineapple chunks or chewing gum. Drowsiness or confusion and respiratory depression (see page 212) can be troublesome, especially in older people, but the symptoms settle once the morphine dose has remained the same for a few days.

Most of the anti-inflammatory drugs have side effects, in particular the NSAID group. They work by inhibiting certain enzyme activity, but as they cannot be selective in their action, they also block enzymes vital to the protection of the lining in the stomach and small intestine. You will be advised about appropriate measures at the time of prescribing; for example, to take dietary precautions or an anti-acid type medication. If certain drugs cause too many unpleasant side effects the doctor can prescribe an alternative medication that is just as effective.

Becoming addicted

Fear of addiction is a commonly expressed worry by patients and their relatives; however, in reality, the possibility is very slight. The dose of any painkilling drug is carefully worked out and monitored to control the pain, until the next dose is due. It relates directly to the level of pain and should not be associated with the severity of the illness. Doctors will start patients off on a low to medium dose and increase it according to need. Differing pain threshold levels are taken into account by careful and accurate pain assessment, the key to getting the levels correct. Tell the doctor honestly how you feel because, if the medication is not controlling the pain, the dose may need to be increased or supplemented with a second drug.

The following descriptions should help to explain some terms in common use.

- **Addiction** This word refers to psychological dependency, typified by an overpowering desire for the drug. The reason why drug addicts become addicted and crave larger doses is because they are pursuing increased levels of drug-induced pleasure; they are not using the drug to ease pain. The risk of addiction from taking opium-based medication for pain relief is very low.

- **Tolerance** This term is used to cover the state when a person gets accustomed to a drug and will probably require a higher dose to maintain comfortable pain control. The raising of the dosage does not mean that tolerance to a particular drug group is likely to cause problems. Usually, the need for an increased dose is because the pain level has risen for physical reasons, rather than higher tolerance developing to the drug.

- **Dependence** This expression is used to describe the physical reliance that a person has on a drug. If dose levels are not maintained, or the drug is withdrawn abruptly, distressing symptoms may appear very quickly and, in the case of opium-based drugs, after only a short period of use. However, because higher doses of opium-type drugs are prescribed primarily to relieve intense pain in a potentially terminal illness, it is very unlikely that the drug administration would be changed. With other types of drugs, such as tranquillisers, where symptoms of dependency are well documented following too fast a withdrawal, doctors take great care to wean patients off their medication at a comfortably tapering rate.

For more information

- CancerBACUP booklet *Feeling better: controlling pain and other symptoms* (see page 203 for address).

- The Pain Relief Foundation leaflet *Cancer Pain* (see page 208 for address).

Non-drug techniques

Many non-drug therapies work well and go a long way towards relieving mild to moderate pain. The options are plentiful and so are the ways in which they can be employed; examples include, sole use or in combination with drug treatments, or as complementary therapies available as home-based products or from a pain clinic, the doctor's surgery or health centre or independent practitioners, and so on. Some treatments, traditionally regarded as complementary or alternative, have now become sufficiently mainstream to have their own entries in this section.

Note: the following list is written in alphabetical order for convenience only; the order in which the techniques appear has no bearing on their value as treatments.

Chiropractic

Chiropractors work in a very similar way to osteopaths (see page 134) to help correct disorders in joints and muscles, especially the area around the spine such as lower back and neck pain. Whiplash injury (see page 82) is a very common reason for many people to visit a chiropractor. Pain emanating from spinal problems can have far reaching effects, causing discomfort in limbs and joints including, the shoulders, hips and legs. Chiropractic relies on the skilful use of hand manipulation and, like osteopathy does not use drugs or surgery; however, a chiropractor would make far more use of conventional diagnostic procedures – such as X-rays – than an osteopath might.

Cognitive behaviour therapy (CBT)

The main aim of *behavioural forms* of therapy is to help people 'learn to believe in themselves' by boosting their self-confidence. It is a form of psychotherapy that works to alter the perceptions, memories and thoughts of people who have a bad feeling about something relating to themselves. This could include any number of past experiences, so each person's reason for feeling that way, and the healing therapy undertaken, will be unique to them. For example, one person could have a heightened perception of pain which in turn affects their interpretation of their actual pain level. For another person, unpleasant memories about the traumatic accident that caused the pain might bring on frightening panic attacks when they attempt to drive a car. Some psychotherapists believe that negative thoughts engender negative beliefs, so thought processes in connection with pain could be stuck in a self-perpetuating, harmful cycle. This in turn could cloud judgement about other aspects of life. The therapy attempts to reverse this process by encouraging people to think and act positively. CBT was first introduced to the arena of psychotherapy in the 1960s by an American psychologist and is a well-known form of treatment which may be arranged by a GP or offered at a pain clinic.

Complementary therapies

Several well-tried treatments can be used to ease aches and pains; for example, acupuncture and acupressure, aromatherapy, massage and hypnotherapy (including self-hypnosis). Most are very straightforward and the simpler methods can be tried at home. (See Chapter 5 for a range of non-orthodox therapies.)

Counselling

Talking to a trained counsellor about anxieties and fears surrounding pain may help reduce stress levels and improve your feelings about the disease. Counselling-type therapy can be less formal than psychotherapy and often takes a practical approach to helping clients deal with problems. Counselling usually helps people focus on their main worries, so they can best solve those problems that can be tackled and move forward in their lives. The counsellor asks questions, listens to the responses and helps the person come to terms with any difficulties that cannot be resolved. If it becomes apparent that anxiety about the pain is linked to other problems, the counsellor may recommend that you visit another agency which can provide very specialist counselling. For example, a counsellor working for a disease-related charity, such as Arthritis Care or the National Back Pain Association, could help a client accept that what they are feeling is a form of grieving for their lost health and that it can never be restored to its former physical state. Counselling would also be available to help focus on issues that might have arisen as a direct result of coping with a chronic illness, for example, with a relationship or alcohol dependency.

Counselling is usually viewed as a shorter-term measure, and counsellors may know early on whether the client is responding to their help and support. Ask a practice or specialist pain nurse how to arrange counselling or contact a national charity helpline (see page 201 for a list of addresses and telephone numbers) for support with a specific disorder. Talking to people who are close to you, such as family members, relatives or friends, is also very beneficial and someone may be able to recommend a local, private counsellor. However, before you involve a person whom you know well, read the advice given in the section 'Finding support' on page 148 so that you are aware of the need to set boundaries.

The British Association for Counselling and Psychotherapy publishes a directory of counsellors in the UK (address on page 202).

Distraction

The act of concentrating on something engrossing can help to take the mind off the symptoms and reduce the tiring effect of pain. Use well tested examples, such as listening to music or a talking tape, reading and watching television. It is also worth trying alternative methods, such as visualisation and relaxation techniques (see pages 149–152) that are easy to learn at home.

The Expert Patients Programme

The 'Expert Patients Programme' is an initiative available through the NHS. It is designed to enable people who have a chronic health condition to gain greater control over their lives by learning how to understand and manage their illness. Taking part in the course helps people increase their knowledge and skills, feel more confident and be more in charge of their lives. For example, 'expert patients' will be helped to communicate more effectively, work in partnership with health care professionals and share responsibility for planning their treatment. The programme also encourages people to be realistic about the full impact their condition might have on their personal lives, and on the lives of the people around them.

Expert patient courses are led by people who themselves have a long term health condition. Each course lasts for six weeks, with two half-hour sessions per week. To find out more telephone 0845 606 6040 or visit the website (see page 205).

Nerve blocks

This technique works by blocking the pain 'messages' that travel along the nerve pathways. Several methods are used which all aim to relieve and control chronic pain, for example:

* long acting local anaesthetics injected into the site;

* cryotherapy (freezing technique);

* heat therapy (radiofrequency thermo-coagulation technique);

* surgical removal of the nerve.

These procedures can be accessed only via the medial services and are part of the key range of therapies offered by pain clinics. A clear explanation of the technique to be applied would be given prior to the treatment.

William's story

William is in his early seventies, and has suffered from intermittent back pain due to a trapped sciatic nerve for many years. For several years he was also the main carer for his wife who was housebound following a stroke. William is an enthusiastic amateur artist, and fortunately was able to arrange for someone to come in and sit with his wife one afternoon a week, so he could go to his art classes. He described this as 'a real lifesaver'. William has lived alone since being widowed five years ago.

When William's back is bad he cannot paint, because he cannot stand at an easel. He can feel very low at such times because isolation and frustration seem to intensify his experience of the physical pain.

For many years, William 'coped' with a combination of over-the-counter painkillers (specifically ibuprofen), physiotherapy and, at times of particular difficulty, a variety of different painkilling drugs prescribed by his doctor. Ten years ago, he was referred to a pain clinic for the first time. It was the pain clinic that recommended long-acting local anaesthetic to be given by epidural injection. William said at the time: 'It was amazing – like getting my life back. I hadn't realised how much I'd lost while the pain was so bad all the time.'

William's first injection lasted for about nine months and the procedure has been repeated several times since. He still has periods of acute pain, but he finds he copes much better knowing that relief is possible. 'At least I know they can do something now' he says. 'It makes such a difference.'

Osteopathy

Osteopathy is one of the most widely practised of all the complementary forms of medicine. It focuses on the skeletal system (joints, muscles and ligaments) and aims to diagnose and treat any mechanical problems affecting the body framework. The two most common reasons for problems developing within the skeletal framework are injury and stress. Any discomfort following an injury may be immediate or it may develop much later. (Here the term 'stress' is used in a technical sense rather like over-bending a piece of metal, and not as an emotional outcome). Trained osteopaths use their hands to massage and manipulate areas of the body to help restore normal function and in doing so relieve any causal pain. Osteopathy is used particularly for problems arising from a malfunction of the spinal cord; to treat various sports-related injuries; osteoarthritis which tends to affect older people, and the type of tension headache commonly caused by the contraction of muscles at the base of the skull.

Physiotherapy

Physiotherapy aims to treat painful conditions and encourage rehabilitation by harnessing the power and benefits of natural forces; for example, physiotherapists work with sources of heat, light and electricity and are experienced in massage, manipulation and remedial exercises. They can advise on how to set goals in pain management, how to relax and how to sleep better. A physiotherapist is likely to play a key role in any treatment prescribed at a pain clinic and they can also be accessed in the community through a surgery or health centre or private practice; where necessary home treatment can be arranged.

Posture and position

Make sure your body is positioned comfortably so that muscles, joints and scar tissue are not being stretched beyond their natural limits. During the day change position regularly to ease pressure and relax muscles. Try a different chair if well-used furniture has become less comfortable and use aids such as sheepskins and pillows to give support if long periods are spent sitting relatively immobile.

If your body is already feeling tired and strained, any movements that increase muscular tension can be an extra drain on your energy reserves so it is worth being as relaxed as possible. Ask a friend to observe your general posture or catch sight of yourself in the mirror or a shop window. Look out for uncomfortable positions and bad habits, such as:

- head thrusting forward or bent down with your chin hard on your chest;
- shoulders hunched and rounded;
- arms held tightly across your chest or stiffly by your sides with hands clenched;
- legs crossed over and twined together;
- restless habits such as tapping fingers and feet, or hair twisting;
- nail biting and teeth clenching.

Consider purchasing a special mattress that helps to induce more restful and comfortable sleep. There is some debate about whether a firmly sprung mattress (sometimes labelled as 'orthopaedic') is in fact the most beneficial structure to ease painful back and joint pains. It has been shown (including at NHS hospitals) that mattresses that mould to the exact shape and position of the body offer the best sleeping posture. The material used in a body-moulding mattress is made from a heat-sensitive, visco-elastic composition, similar to that developed to protect astronauts from the G-force experienced during accelerated lift-off. The special features developed in this material distribute pressure evenly across the entire contact area, between the body and the mattress, qualities that a standard sprung mattress may not provide. Visco-elastic-type mattresses are readily available through high street stores or by mail-order.

For more information

- Aids and equipment: the local branches of the British Red Cross and St John Ambulance give advice and arrange the hire or loan of equipment – look in the telephone directory for a local number or ask at your surgery or health centre; you may need a referral from a doctor or community nurse for some pieces of equipment.

- *The Back Pain Book,* by Mike Hage, Revised 2nd edition. Class Publishing.

Radiotherapy

This treatment is used to treat pain in bones and some other sites, particularly with cancer patients. Low doses only are necessary to achieve very effective results. The therapy takes about seven to ten days to start working, so other painkillers will need to be taken until the benefits are felt. It may then be possible to reduce the dosage of stronger medication. This therapy can only be accessed through a medical practitioner.

Temperature

Changing the external body temperature can have a very comforting effect. There are several contributing factors that back the reasoning. It is probable that *warmth* to the skin closes the pain gateway, by encouraging the 'feel-good' sensation derived from mental and physical relaxation. Raising the body temperature increases the blood supply to the damaged tissue and promotes healing (but a word of warning – heat should not be applied immediately after an injury has occurred as it could increase the swelling). Heat, for example from a warm bath, loosens up the synovial fluid so arthritic joints may benefit from warmth at the start of the day. *Cold* therapy works best as a first aid treatment immediately following an accident. Plunging burnt tissue directly into very cold water (for at least ten minutes) halts the penetration of heat damage to the deeper, subcutaneous layers and helps to ease the pain. Likewise, soaking a sprained ankle in cold water promptly causes the blood vessels to constrict, which reduces the inflammation and limits further bruising and tissue damage.

Sinead is a physiotherapist
'Warmth and movement are great healing aids. For a self-help approach try a "wheat bag" (available from some pharmacies and health stores, or over the Internet). Its gentle effect can never be over-used or cause undue harm provided a few basic rules are observed; for example, heat should not be applied to the area close to the eyes nor where there are obvious signs of acute inflammation or infection.' (See page 36)

Sometimes, alternating warm and cold brings effective relief. The best method to facilitate the hot or cold therapy can be determined by the temperature required and the length of time that the body part should remain in contact with the heat source. Obvious examples include, putting a limb under running tap water or in a bowl; full immersion in a bath; placing the heat/cold source next to the skin using either a rubber hot water bottle, or a gel-filled container that can be warmed in a microwave oven or cooled in a refrigerator, or an ice pack that can be made from crushed cubes, or substituted with a bag of peas or a 'freezer' container used in cool boxes. For safety as well as comfort always wrap ice packs or similar in a towel to avoid damaging the skin.

TENS machine

The full name for this device is a 'Transcutaneous Electrical Nerve Stimulator'. It can be used to stimulate nerves reaching the brain to encourage the body to produce natural painkillers, chemicals called endorphins. The TENS effect may also help to close the gateway to a part of the brain called the thalamus, where various nerve endings for pain and sensation converge before moving forward to their final 'interpretation' centres. The mild, electrical stimulation is given through adhesive pads placed on the skin surface. It feels like a prickly, tingling sensation, which is rather pleasant. The technique works in a similar way to acupuncture and can be applied to various types of pain, especially that coming from aching joints and muscles, neuralgia and the phantom pain from a previously amputated limb. The small, battery-operated machine can be carried easily in a pocket and there appear to be no adverse side effects. A professional person, such as a physiotherapist or a registered private practitioner, would advise on proper use if you are unsure, as it is important to follow the instructions correctly. The equipment is readily obtainable and can be purchased from most pharmacies, health shops or by mail order. Or ask for information at your GP surgery or specialist pain clinic, or from a physiotherapist.

For more information
* The Pain Relief Foundation leaflet *Electrical stimulators* (see page 208 for address).

Pain management units – eg 'INPUT'

INPUT is a specialist pain management unit at St Thomas' Hospital, London catering for people from all over the UK. It is included here as an example, as several other such units exist around the country. They vary in accessibility, can often have long waiting times and funding may or may not be available from your local Primary Care Trust. On average, the people receiving treatment at specialist pain management units have endured chronic pain for ten years or more and have usually tried many other remedies, without lasting results. Information available on the INPUT website suggests that 'Once pain has been present for more than a year, an operation or drug seldom cures it'.

INPUT offers patients access to a complete pain management programme, in groups of ten people of mixed age and sex; and who are suffering a range of pain problems. The programmes differ in length, with most people staying for either four days per week, for two or four consecutive weeks, or for eight days, over a six-week period. Many other centres offer non-residential places. The residential accommodation at INPUT is in a modern building overlooking the Thames, by Westminster Bridge. Patients stay in comfortably furnished, individual rooms so privacy is assured. The pain management programme is intensive, running from 8.30am to 5.00pm each day. It takes place in the same building as the sleeping accommodation, on the ground floor, where a lounge, conservatory and garden area add to the pleasant surroundings.

The programme aims to teach pain management techniques that will 'become a way of life for the chronic pain sufferer just as a person with diabetes has to take insulin'. The programme is thorough but realistic, and success is more about measuring quality of life than actual cure. Most people report major improvements in their physical capabilities, their mood and their mental state. The programme offers a range of psychological techniques, practical strategies and information sessions, to help patients:

- regain increased mobility and fitness;
- plan, regulate and pace their rate of progress;
- set and achieve certain goals;
- break old habits associated with previous pain control;
- relax muscle tension.

If you think that time spent at a residential specialist pain management unit might help you to manage your pain more efficiently, speak to your hospital consultant or family doctor, who must write a letter of referral. For INPUT, they will need to write to: The Consultant Anaesthetist and Medical Director (see page 205 for address).

Anthea's story

Anthea has a condition known as hypermobility syndrome, an inherited collagen disorder and spinal deformities. The effects of this syndrome have been noticeable for most of her life. Anthea says on bad days she feels extreme exhaustion on top of generalised pain, making it difficult to do anything at all – even watching television is difficult. The pain is generally felt most severely in her spine, which is hyper- (excessively) mobile causing stress in the lower part of her back, chest and neck, often at different times. The pain is sometimes acute and sometimes her muscles go into spasm. Pain occurs throughout the remainder of her body with varying intensity due to frailty of the tissues.

On good days all this pain feels minimal. Over the years Anthea believes she has become less affected by the emotional aspect of the discomfort.

For Anthea the three key words that spring to mind in relation to her illness are 'challenging', 'persistent' and 'recurrent'. Ultimately Anthea feels that there is an element of 'healing' in the sense that the challenge evokes a new 'me'.

In Anthea's case the pain, fortunately, does not affect other people.

The treatment(s) that have worked best for Anthea over the years have been a combination of medication and therapies from the following lists:

Prescribed by the general practitioner or hospital consultant
- *Non-steroidal anti-inflammatory/analgesic drug (Naprosyn) – which she uses only when the pain is unbearable, and it does not always work.*
- *Pain relief (Migraleve) – as she has not tried to face a migraine using mind techniques (yet).*

Self-help treatments
- *Gradually Anthea has come to use an approach which works well for her – to look straight at the pain when it occurs – instead of trying to get on with life by denying it and suppressing any reaction to it, as she did in the past. It does take time and discipline to face the pain but she feels that it 'dismantles' the suffering and releases the energy formerly tied up in suppression and denial. Generally, this technique makes it much easier to live with.*

Complementary therapies
- *Osteopathy*
- *Healing.*

Anthea has been along to a pain clinic where she was interviewed but it was agreed that the above approach was working better than anything that the clinic staff could offer. Certainly, she believes that she is a completely different person since adopting the approach – now a person with symptoms rather than someone lost in a pool of pain symptoms. The process is refining itself all the time and its effects are cumulative.

Conclusion

Relief from pain is achievable. However, there are no miraculous cures and controlling pain takes time. Be realistic in your aims, be focused in your approach and be prepared to try a range of treatments. Drug therapy is likely to figure highly in your treatment programme but not necessarily as a lifelong chore. There are likely to be many other options, depending on the nature of your illness, including self-help and complementary therapies. The next chapter looks at stress relief and at some of the non-orthodox therapies that are readily available for those people who wish to explore them.

5 Stress relief and non-orthodox treatments

Feeling unwell is stressful for many reasons. The overriding physical presence of pain, anxieties about the future, and the extra pressures of trying to manage your life generally all contribute towards emotional and physical fatigue. It is no wonder most people with chronic pain say that feelings of tension rarely go away.

This chapter describes the main elements of stress and helps you focus on your personal problems. How you deal with a difficult situation depends on all sorts of factors – your personality type, how much control you feel, and how much energy you have in reserve. All can play their part in your ability to cope.

Everyone needs a few strategies to draw upon when it is important to be mentally strong or reduce tension. This chapter looks at ways to build up your personal strengths and develop some support systems. It offers a selection of coping skills to use when you feel at the end of your tether, yet need to remain calm. Relaxing your muscles or enjoying an aromatherapy massage can work wonders when you are feeling pressured and over-tired. You also need to find agreeable ways to protect yourself from the traumas of everyday living. This chapter helps you to do that by looking at some of the therapies and treatments that can be used alongside orthodox medicine to treat stress as part of a pain management programme. It describes some of the popular complementary treatments such as aromatherapy, reflexology, homeopathy and massage, and suggests how you and a partner or relative might benefit. Some can easily be practised at home using basic remedies and techniques but, for others, it would be advisable to see a qualified practitioner.

What is 'stress'?

The word 'stress' is very popular nowadays, and is commonly used to describe the way we feel when pressure is intense. It is not a medical problem but a combination of symptoms produced when our physical, mental and emotional systems go into overdrive. Everyone's body reacts to stress in the same physical way, whatever the cause or size of the problem. Unfortunately, though, some people seem to get more upset than others when faced by difficult situations. This stronger reaction to stress is often produced by a combination of factors – the person's emotional state at the time, their inherent personality type and how well they have learned to cope in the past – rather than the extent of the problem.

High stress levels for people in pain are likely to stem from:

- the unremitting discomfort;
- lack of sleep;
- feeling that your illness is not within your control;
- difficult relationships and pressures from other people;
- lack of knowledge;
- low morale;
- uncertainty about the future.

Primitive feelings

Coping with day-to-day stress is normal because a small amount of pressure can improve performance. It keeps your brain stimulated and helps you concentrate and deal with challenging situations. For example, many performers regard a bit of stress as essential: it adds sparkle to their act and keeps them alert. But when the pressure becomes too great, the physical reaction can be unpleasant. As tension builds up, your body produces high levels of the hormone adrenaline to prepare itself for action in the same way as a primitive caveman. This reaction, known as the 'fight or flight' mechanism, enabled him to respond swiftly to danger. For us, however, unlike our ancestors, this type of 'escape' is rarely necessary. So instead of using up the energy generated to deal with the hazard (stressful situation) it remains in the system, keeping it in a continual state of tension. While adrenaline levels are high, you probably feel as if you are living on the edge of a crisis so it takes little additional worry to make you feel very anxious. The tension can become so intense that you may feel as if you are about to explode and you can no longer handle all of the demands being made of you. If you 'listen' to your body it is telling you that it feels extremely distressed.

Warning signs

The signs and symptoms that indicate that you might be feeling over-stressed are triggered by a combination of physical and emotional re-actions. Look at the list below and note the ones that trouble you regu-larly. The symptoms of stress may or may not be closely associated with an existing illness. If you are bothered by more than a few the time is right to consider some solutions before your health is damaged further:

- headaches;

- increase in pain;

- listlessness and fatigue;

- difficulty in sleeping at either end of the night;

- palpitations and rapid pulse rate;

- indigestion or heartburn;

- breathing problems (particularly if breathing becomes faster and more shallow);

- eating too much or not enough;

- skin problems;

- increased need to pass urine, and nervous diarrhoea;

- numbness or pins and needles in limbs;

- poor concentration and difficulty making decisions;

- feeling unhappy and depressed;

- feeling angry, frustrated and helpless;

- feeling irritable and tearful;

- anxiety and fearfulness;

- loss of sense of humour.

Where do all the stresses come from?

It is difficult to define stress clearly because it feels as if it comes from two directions, both external and internal. The confusion arises when we talk about stress as a cause of problems (pressures from people or situations) and as an effect (a response from inside our bodies, such as a severe migraine). Both internal and external stresses affect our moods and the physical ability to cope. Unfortunately, not all sources of stress are within our control, and problems can rarely be packaged neatly into distinct 'causes'. Mostly we manage to keep the troubles isolated and give our bodies sufficient rest before dealing with the next set of problems. But when you are already dealing with pain this may not always be possible.

Psychologists refer to these sources of stress as 'life events' and they include major upheavals like retirement, moving home, changing job, an accident and illness but also lesser events such as Christmas or going on holiday. They aren't particularly special or rare, and they aren't necessarily unpleasant – just things that happen to all of us all of the time. However, if a string of events happen too close together, pressure builds up to uncomfortable levels and it takes only one small problem to bring everything to a head. The important point to note is that it is the accumulation of both major and minor events coming together that creates the worse scenario, rather than merely the severity of the events.

Stress triggers

If the build-up of tension has already reached a critical level, it won't take much to tip you over the top. Do the following 'nerve janglers' seem familiar?

- Tiredness caused by insufficient sleep due to frequent interruptions in the night, or altered sleep patterns such as waking early.

- Prolonged pain perhaps from the continual physical strain produced by aching joints.

- Fragile emotions stemming from anger or anxiety about your ill health.

- Frustration and pressures created by people or places – demanding lifestyle, hospital appointments, shopping in crowded supermarkets.

- Discomfort caused by lack of fresh air, too much noise or feeling too hot or too cold.

- Depressing weather – some people are adversely affected by too little sunlight and long dark evenings.

- Sensitive digestive system – the side effects from long-term drug treatments, too much alcohol, caffeine in tea and coffee or refined sugar can all exacerbate stress.

- Craving for a cigarette because anxiety levels are high. Stress is the reason many people give for continuing to smoke.

- Uncertainty about the future and possible financial worries.

- Impatient personality – some people tend to be quicker to react than others.

Getting the balance right

The key to managing stress is getting the balancing act right between tension and relaxation – like a juggler if you get too many plates in the air at once they all come crashing down. Being ill can bring extra respon-sibilities. If you are the main person your family relies on, balancing your own needs against theirs may be hard to achieve. Unfortunately, you are the one most likely to end up with too much stress and too little time for relaxation. Tension and anxiety can't be switched off to order but this does not mean they should be ignored, as being over-stressed can lead to depression. There are ways to ease the pressure and give your body a rest, and stress is easier to bear if you understand and accept where the problems are coming from. Try not to be 'superhuman'. Think about what jobs need tackling and divide them into those that are urgent and those that can wait. It is amazing how the mind clears when the priorities have been sorted out.

John had multiple fractures following an accident
'I had to learn very swiftly to adjust to being helped. For a few weeks my wife had to do everything for me. Either she anticipated my needs or I had to ask for help. Not being able to move my arms made me very nervous as I worried constantly about falling over.'

Stress diary

Writing a stress diary can help to sort out how you feel. It may seem like yet another task but a few minutes spent now may save you from sleepless hours later (see also pain diary, page 112). Start the process by making a list of all the things that have bothered you in the last week. Next jot down by the side of each problem how you felt at the time – angry, anxious, irritable, etc. Now circle the things that you chose to do willingly – they may have been difficult, but if you accept their importance you are less likely to be upset by the effort. Look at the remainder of the problems on your list and ask yourself if they could be the cause of your increased anxiety. Are they stemming from external pressure or internal worries over which you have little control? The reason why many people get angry and upset about some situations and not others is often linked to their feelings about choice. Can you cross anything off your list to ease the pressure?

Mental stimulation

Stress doesn't always arise from over-activity. It is also possible to feel frustrated and unsettled if you are bored, isolated at home and repeating the same routine day after day – a scenario which might sound familiar to someone whose pain prevents them from being as active as they would wish. It is unrealistic to believe you can exercise control over every aspect of your life, but at least try to manage your free time to counteract the daily turmoil. For example, if there is pressure at home or pain levels are high, choose a relaxing pastime. Don't take on extra responsibilities outside of the house, or engage in strenuous activities. If you are isolated at home, arrange to spend respite time in pleasant company, perhaps involving some interesting conversation.

Helping yourself

By now you will probably have gained a clearer picture about the main causes of your stress and feel ready to make some changes that will help you to cope. Start the process by asking yourself how you dealt with difficult situations in the past and what lessons you learned from that process. Then think about what is different this time round, and what steps might be needed to help you get along. Remember that problems are rarely solved in isolation so think about who (or what) you could turn to for support. Finally, accept that not all problems can be 'solved'. Your illness may not disappear entirely, but you can do your best to deal with it in the best way possible.

Finding ways to cope with pressure

No one ever 'cured' their stress overnight – so don't rush into hasty decisions. Look at each problem separately with four courses of action in mind:

- **One** Is it necessary to change the situation? This course may call for major action, such as moving into more suitable accommodation, perhaps without stairs. Making a decision of this nature will be extremely upsetting so do not attempt to make it alone. But if you are finding it very difficult to cope, it could be the right solution in the longer term.

- **Two** Can you improve your ability to deal with the situation? Your stress levels might fall quite dramatically if you ease some of the pressure on yourself and your time. A practical solution, such as getting help with the housework, could be the answer.

- **Three** Do you need to change your perception of the situation? Ask yourself whether the problem is as bad as you think it is (either the immediate problem that's worrying you right now or the longer term effects of the illness) and try to turn some of the threats into challenges. Positive 'self-talk' works well here: tell yourself that you have dealt with difficult situations before and that you have ample reserves of inner strength.

- **Four** Would changing your routine help? Doing things through habit is easy, especially if you are feeling upset, but your routine may be increasing your stress and your pain. If you are forcing yourself to be busy, slow down so that your actions become calmer. This gives your brain a less-stressed message. Learn how to pace yourself, as this is a major factor in pain management. Cut down on the amount of coffee and tea you drink – the caffeine they contain stimulates the nervous system causing irritability and insomnia. Change any routines that are particularly tiring; for example, avoid shopping at busy times and make use of the customer facilities offered by many supermarkets, such as home delivery or goods carried to your car.

Personal resources

Draw up a list of your strengths and personal resources that you really value. You might include some of the following examples:

- firm relationships with a partner, children, family and friends;
- a positive mental attitude and inner confidence;
- pleasure from your job or hobbies;
- a sense of humour;
- financial security;
- spiritual support;
- non-dependence on smoking, alcohol or drugs.

In a similar way you could think about where you feel vulnerable. Identify situations where it may be possible to improve your ability to cope – for example, by:

- learning to reduce the pressure you impose on yourself;
- having the confidence to say 'no' sometimes;
- delegating to others some of the household jobs that are difficult to manage.

You may find it helpful to talk to someone you trust about the steps you could take to improve the areas where you feel insecure, at least to the point where you feel less anxious. Take each step gently; this is not a time to push yourself.

Finding support

Any support is valuable when you are feeling under pressure, especially if it is undemanding. Asking for help is not a sign of weakness; it is more a demonstration of awareness that problems can seldom be solved alone. If you are beginning to feel depressed yourself it is vital you seek help. You may need to make the first move with friends and relatives by asking for a listening ear, as they may be reticent about 'interfering' unless invited. Once you have given the signal to initiate help, you should discuss with the other person how this can be achieved without upsetting your relationship. It is important to agree a few basic rules at the beginning, because the last thing you want is someone marching in and taking over. For example, the person you talk to must respect your need for confidentiality; and they need to be aware that you may become emotional and let off a 'bit of steam'. Also, you must feel free to ignore their advice without fear of causing offence.

If talking to a friend or relative is not the best course for you (because you would find this uncomfortable or there isn't a suitable person) other options are available. Ask your doctor or the practice nurse, or the pain clinic staff, if they can recommend a professional person or group. If you choose a private counsellor be sure they are trained and registered. Consider any of the following sources of support:

- a therapist who specialises in stress or psychological counselling or cognitive therapy;

- a self-help support network;

- a religious leader or other form of spiritual support;

- a telephone helpline (eg many health charities offer some type of verbal support);

- the Samaritans (the national 24-hour helpline staffed by trained counsellors who offer emotional support to people who are feeling isolated and in despair – 08457 90 90 90 or see local telephone directory).

Learning to relax

Better breathing

Breathing is an unconscious action that you rarely think about, but over the years you may have developed poor breathing habits without realising their significance. Irregular breathing patterns, such as hyperventilation or overbreathing, can increase anxiety levels. When your body is calm, breathing is slow, regular and deep. But when anxiety levels are high the opposite happens, breathing becomes fast, irregular and shallow, creating feelings of panic. Breathing is normally controlled by the involuntary nervous system but it is possible to take control of the process and calm the system down when pressure begins to rise. People who learn to breathe calmly when they are feeling tense soon notice an improvement in their anxiety state. The following guidelines will help you to correct overbreathing and generally reduce tension:

- As soon as anxiety levels begin to rise, quietly tell yourself to 'calm down'. This sends a positive message to the brain.

- Slow down all your movements, because rushing around increases agitation and your body responds by producing more adrenaline to deal with the 'threat'.

- Calm your breathing deliberately and keep an even rhythm with a slight pause between the in and out breaths; imagine a candle in front of your face which gently flickers as you breathe out.

- Practise calm breathing at different times during the day so that you are aware of the feeling of taking control. It is much easier to recognise the correct pattern when you are not over anxious.

Deep relaxation

Deep relaxation is an excellent way to restore energy and boost your spirits, but it does need time and space. Merely telling yourself to relax is unlikely to work, especially if you are feeling overwrought. Relaxation is easy to learn but it does require practice. It may take several sessions to get it right and it helps if you understand how the technique works. It is all about fooling the system and giving out positive signals that your body is at ease. Relaxed muscles and slow, quiet breathing send calming messages to the brain that turns off the false reaction to danger. When there are no threats your body rests and restores itself, ready for the next burst of energy.

Whole body relaxation

This is the most common form of relaxation and produces pleasant results quickly. The technique works better if you create the right conditions and allow sufficient time – about twenty minutes for a whole body session. Eventually, you can cut down on the time and recreate the stress-free feeling anywhere as you improve your skill. If you would like to learn to relax with a teacher, ask at your GP surgery or health centre. Many stress counsellors run individual or group classes.

Step by step technique for use at home

1   Find a warm, quiet place and lie on a rug or sit in a well supported chair. Use a pillow for support if it helps to make you more comfortable. Reduce outside noises if possible.

2   Wear loose clothing and remove glasses and shoes. Lie on your back with your head supported, and your arms and legs straight

and slightly apart. If you are sitting, put your feet flat on the floor and have your knees slightly apart.

3   Breathe in and out deeply for three breaths and imagine you are loosening the tension. Then breathe normally.

4   You can close your eyes at this stage or wait until they shut naturally. You are going to work on each major muscle group starting with the feet. As you tighten and relax the muscles learn to recognise the difference between tension and relaxation. Hold each contraction for a few seconds and repeat each action with a short break between.

5   Pull your feet towards your body – hold the tension – release and feel the reduction in tension.

6   Point your toes hard away from your body and feel the tension in your calf muscles – hold – and relax.

7   Next work on your thighs by drawing your legs tightly towards you or raising them into the air – hold – drop back to a relaxed position with thighs rolled outwards.

8   Tense your buttocks by squeezing them hard together – hold – and relax.

9   Tense your abdomen in the opposite way by pushing it outwards – hold – and then let it flop.

10   Check your legs again and if you have slipped back into a tense position have a second go from Step 5. A couple of deep breaths will help at this point. Your lower body should feel heavy, warm and relaxed.

11   Now concentrate on your back. Arch your spine away from the floor or chair – hold – and relax. (**Warning:** leave this one out if you have any back problems.)

12   Now move your shoulders backwards to expand your chest – hold – and relax.

13   Tense your shoulders next by raising your arms and pulling on your shoulders – hold – as you drop your arms wriggle your shoulders up to your ears and relax with your shoulderblades touching the floor or chair.

14 Now work on your hands and lower arms by making a tight fist – hold – and relax letting your fingers droop. As you clench your fists for the second time raise your arms slightly and notice the tension in your forearms – hold – and relax.

15 Move to the upper arms by bringing your hands across your body, close to your chest – hold – relax them to a position on the floor or beside you with the palms facing upwards.

16 Relax your neck and throat by gently moving your head from side to side (not a circular movement) and then pulling your chin down to your chest – hold – and relax.

17 Next clench your jaw by clamping your teeth together – hold – and let go so that your mouth is slightly open. That tension probably felt familiar as clenching teeth is a common habit.

18 Now work on your facial muscles. Press your lips together – hold – and relax. Push your tongue hard to the roof of your mouth – hold – and let it drop to the floor of your mouth.

19 Move your eyes inside your closed lids to the four quarters of a circle and then let your eyelids relax.

20 Finally relax your forehead and scalp. Frown hard and pull your forehead down – hold – and let go so that your face feels loose.

Your whole body should now feel comfortable and free from tension. Breathe gently and let your mind wander at will. If stressful thoughts irritate you in this relaxed state, think about somewhere pleasant and, as you breathe, repeat in your mind, 'peace in and pressure out'. Don't worry if you drop off to sleep at this point. Eventually you will learn to relax your body without going to sleep, but use this method at night if insomnia is a problem.

Lie quietly with your eyes closed for a few minutes enjoying the warm feeling; then slowly bring yourself back to the present. Count backwards from five to one, clench your fists tightly, relax and rub your hands together. If you are lying on the floor roll onto your side; open your eyes with your hands shielding them from the light. Stand up slowly and try to hold on to the relaxed mood when you return to action.

Getting the best from relaxation

It can be enjoyable to share your relaxation session with another person. You can take turns to read the instructions or make yourselves a tape-recording. Listen to music if it helps to calm your mind and ring the changes by starting at the top and working towards your feet. As you become better at 'switching off', shorten the session and create a relaxed mood by imagining your body is warm and heavy without going through all of the muscle tightening steps. Use this shortened version as a mini-restorative, particularly when you are away from home in stressful situations.

For more information

Addresses can be found in the 'Useful addresses' section (pages 201–210):

- British Association for Counselling and Psychotherapy publishes a directory of counsellors in the UK.

- Family Doctor Series of booklets: *Understanding Stress,* available from most pharmacies.

- Music tapes: *The Fairy Ring* and *Silver Wings,* both by Mike Rowland, and *Spirit of the Rainforest* by Terry Oldfield are soothing tapes to use for relaxation. They are available from music shops or by catalogue from New World Aurora.

- The Stress Management Training Institute publishes a wide range of materials to help reduce stress: leaflets, audio tapes, books and a newsletter.

- The Royal College of Psychiatrists publishes a range of information for dealing with anxieties, phobias and depression. Send a stamped addressed envelope with your request.

- Unwind Pain and Stress Management publishes a range of materials to help reduce stress: self-help programmes, tapes, books and helpline backup. Send a stamped addressed envelope for details.

Complementary treatments to help manage your pain

The terms 'alternative therapy' and 'complementary therapy' are used to describe a range of treatments available from practitioners and therapists who work to treat the whole body, either alongside, or instead of, treatments offered by conventional medicine. In order to clarify the difference in meaning, the following descriptions are commonly accepted.

- **Conventional medicine** This covers a range of treatments that you may have already received, including medication and orthodox therapies, which have been widely used throughout the world for many years and have undergone expert clinical trials.

- **Unconventional medicine** This covers a number of treatments that are widely used and, on the whole, widely respected. Included in this group are homeopathy and herbal medicine. Practitioners do not claim the medications used will cure pain or stress but the treatments may help to reduce the symptoms caused by the disorder and the side effects of orthodox treatments.

- **Complementary therapies** These are therapies intended for use alongside (as a 'complement' to) orthodox medicine rather than replacing it. Examples could include physical treatments such as aromatherapy and reflexology, and counselling to benefit the person's state of mind. The treatments may be beneficial, as complementary therapies can help to combat tension and stress and give a welcome boost to your morale.

- **Alternative therapies** These therapies are usually held to be treatments that are given *instead* of conventional treatments. These therapies often involve regimens that attempt to treat the illness direct, using non-medical methods. Most alternative therapies have not been subjected to clinical trials.

Many popular complementary treatments originated in the East and have been practised there for centuries. They rely on ancient knowledge linked to herbal remedies and traditional practices that are believed to stimulate the body's own healing powers. Acupuncture from China and yoga from India are obvious examples. Some of the newer therapies appeal more to Western scientific minds and are used as aids to diagnosis as well as treatment. Two examples are colour therapy, that draws links between certain colours and mental harmony or stress, and iridology that examines the eyes for clues to hidden disorders.

All complementary and alternative treatments can be obtained without going to a medically trained doctor, but this does not mean that an NHS or private doctor will not or cannot provide some complementary treatments. Some doctors are dually trained, and many GPs now recommend the benefits of certain therapies. Increasingly, complementary therapies are being introduced into the NHS and are available at day centres and GP practices, either free of charge or with a fee. Geographical location may affect your ability to find a suitable practitioner; ask at your local library, GP surgery or health centre. Be prepared to sample more than one type, as those that work for one person may well not suit another.

A note of caution: before using any complementary or alternative therapy, especially if you are receiving other medication and treatments, it is extremely important to consult your doctor. There are several reasons for seeking advice before starting a non-conventional treatment:

- some therapies use extracts from plants which can have very powerful properties that may affect other treatments;

- the effort of being massaged may be too tiring for you if parts of your body are frail;

- some therapies use methods that have not been scientifically tested;

- some remedies can have an interaction with conventional drugs.

There is some conflict of opinion between supporters of conventional medicine and supporters of alternative therapies. Many doctors providing orthodox treatment are concerned that alternative cures may be harmful. Patients sometimes reject conventional medicine and seek alternative remedies out of a false sense of hope and promises of amazing cures. There is no justifiable evidence that such cures exist, and no reputable therapist would ever make such claims.

It is tempting to think that herbal remedies are completely harmless, but this is not necessarily true. Some professional bodies, for example, the American Food and Drug Administration and the American Society of Anaesthesiologists, warn that many such treatments should be stopped at least two weeks prior to surgery. The same advice would also be relevant in the UK. If you are taking any herbal remedies, you should always mention this both to your surgeon and to your anaesthetist.

Several of the therapies described in this chapter can be practised at home using basic remedies and techniques learned from a book. If you use information from a book to prepare treatment materials be sure to follow the instructions carefully. However, rather than spend time learning new techniques you may prefer to receive treatment from a qualified practitioner.

Finding a qualified therapist

Some complementary therapies cannot be recommended for self-help practice and it is advisable that treatment is obtained only from a trained practitioner. Ask for details of reputable, local therapists at your GP surgery or health centre. Alternatively, you could contact the national organisations listed in the 'For more information' sections or on pages 201–210). Word of mouth can be a good form of recommendation, but do make sure any therapist you visit is registered to practise with the appropriate national body.

Don't be embarrassed to ask directly about qualifications, as all reputable therapists will be pleased to offer reassurance and tell you how to check. Properly trained therapists take a full medical history before prescribing. They will have learned about the effects of the remedies they use, whereas untrained people can only guess and may do harm. There are some ready made treatments available in health shops, but it would be wise to consult a doctor first, before taking any over-the-counter medication, so you do not delay diagnosis or effective orthodox treatment. Finally, whichever complementary or alternative treatment you choose, it is wise to consult a medical doctor if symptoms persist.

You may be sceptical about whether or not a particular therapy works, especially if it relies upon less orthodox and 'unseen' methods. No therapist or practitioner of complementary therapies will ever claim to 'cure' a patient alone, or to replace orthodox medicine. But they would strongly support the notion that their treatments can contribute towards a feeling of well-being. People who use a practitioner can expect to receive more time for treatment, a 'whole body' approach to their problems and advice about self-help. If your health is less robust it is well worth considering some of these treatments, as they can bring tremendous relief from distress and discomfort. Also, spending time receiving individual attention and feeling pampered is likely to help you feel a little better in yourself.

Acupressure

Acupressure is an ancient skill practised in China and Japan for over 3,000 years. It combines massage with the principles of acupuncture (without using needles), and is thought to have been the forerunner of acupuncture. Acupressure is believed to improve the body's healing powers, prevent illness and promote energy. Practitioners work on known pressure points with thumbs, fingertips, palms, elbows, knees and feet to balance the flow of energy called 'chi', which runs through 'meridians' or invisible channels throughout the body. Acupressure relieves the symptoms of many conditions and is best used in conjunction with other natural or orthodox treatments. It is thought to be beneficial with many conditions, especially those in which stress may play a part. Examples include asthma, back pain, depression, insomnia, migraine, and general tension.

Your acupressure therapist will take a full personal history and then use acupressure points to sedate or stimulate the energy channels. Weekly treatments may be needed to improve a problem, or you could just enjoy a regular tone-up to promote well-being. Instructions for 'self-help' acupressure can be taken from a book and practised alone or with a partner. However, it is advisable that only minor everyday problems such as headache or nausea are treated without the expertise of a trained practitioner.

A useful technique to try will help relieve nausea caused by travel sickness or anxiety. This remedy is supported by research at Belfast University's Department of Anaesthesia that has shown that the use of pressure bands (sea bands) worn around the wrists does ease feelings of nausea. Similar studies have concluded that acupressure can help with post-operative nausea and vomiting

Method 1 – for nausea

1   Press with the pad of your thumb on the point (called 'pericardium 6') on the inner wrist, about 5cm (2 inches) from the joint, between the tendons. The pressure should be firm enough to cause some discomfort but not pain.

2   Hold for 5–10 minutes. Repeat as often as necessary.

Method 2 – for headache and facial pains

1 Locate the point ('large intestine 4') by placing the thumb and fore-finger of one hand over the web of skin between the thumb and forefinger of the other hand, slightly towards the index finger.

2 Squeeze firmly for about five minutes. Repeat as often as necessary.

For more information

• To find your nearest practitioner, contact the Council for Complementary and Alternative Medicine (address on page 204) enclosing an SAE.

Acupuncture

Acupuncture shares all the qualities of acupressure and, although its powers are not fully understood, it is fast gaining followers in Western medicine as a credible form of pain management. The technique differs little from acupressure other than that specialist needles are used in place of pressure. Research has shown that the needles stimulate sensory nerves in the skin and muscles, which in turn transmit signals to the spine and brain. The prompt incites pain modulation triggered by the release of endorphins, the body's own opioid substances. In addition, it is probable that pain-blocking and anti-inflammatory chemicals are also released into the bloodstream.

Warning: it is NOT possible to practise acupuncture as a self-help technique; a qualified therapist must ALWAYS be used to avoid the risk of doing serious harm.

Acupuncture is offered by many pain clinics, some physiotherapy departments and from private practitioners.

For more information

• To find your nearest practitioner, contact the British Acupuncture Council (address on page 202).

Aromatherapy

The ancient art of aromatherapy combines the healing properties of aromatic plant essences with massage, and is an excellent therapy to try if complementary treatments are new to you (see note of caution, page 155). It is a gentle method that encourages a relaxed feeling, and a trained therapist will ask questions first to discover the best treatment for each individual person. The complex essential oils extracted from many plants are introduced into the body where the 'life force' of the plant's essential oil can have a beneficial effect. Therapists do not claim that the oils heal directly in the sense that a synthetic drug may effect a cure; rather it is believed that the oils encourage the body to use its own natural healing forces from within. The essential oils are absorbed through the skin and pass through the tissues to the bloodstream and so travel around the body. Different combinations of oils affect different parts of the body – for example, rosemary is recommended for backache and muscular problems.

When buying aromatherapy oils, always choose 'pure essential' oils to ensure good quality. Labels which state 'fragrance' or 'blend' are synthetic and are useful only as mood creators or to scent a room. There are recognised retail outlets in most high streets – try good health food, body care and herbalist shops, pharmacies and the larger supermarkets.

Note of caution: Essential oils are extracted from plant essences by a special distillation process that changes their chemical composition. They are used in concentrations that are many times stronger than their original plant form and are rarely used undiluted because they are too powerful to use directly on the skin. Before use, essential oils should always be mixed with a carrier (or base) oil such as almond or peach oil. It is important to be aware that essential oils are very powerful, and that their use is not advised with people who suffer from certain conditions such as a history of miscarriage, haemophilia, advanced varicose veins or a high temperature. Always read the instructions carefully before use or follow the advice of a qualified therapist. Aromatherapy oils should never be taken by mouth.

Methods for use at home
The soothing oils can be used in several ways to enhance their effect:

- **Vaporisation** This creates a very pleasant effect by burning oils in special containers, so that the aroma is inhaled from the air. It is believed that the healing part of the oil is breathed into the body and passes through the membranes of the lungs into the blood system. Pottery containers and blended oils are readily available in many gift shops. Fill the bowl with water, add 2-4 drops of your chosen oil and place a lighted night-light candle underneath.

- **Blending oils with other creams** This gives extra benefit for skin care to reduce dry skin and enrich hand and body creams. Mix together one drop of chamomile oil, two drops of geranium oil and one drop of lavender oil, with a basic over-the-counter skin cream or 20ml of base oil to make a rich skin preparation.

- **Scented baths** Mix five drops of pure essential oil (such as lavender) with one tablespoon of carrier oil and add to the bathwater to relax the body or ease aching joints. Add other oils (such as sandalwood and ylang-ylang) to promote a restful night's sleep.

- **Inhalation** Use in steam inhalers or place droplets on a handkerchief or pillow to bring relief from colds and chronic catarrh. Three drops of eucalyptus oil and two drops of geranium, mixed into 2.5 mls of base oil, provide an aromatic bath version, instead of the traditional head-steaming method.

- **As an aromatherapy massage** Simple massage techniques (gentler than the vigorous massages given by professional therapists) can easily be learned from instructions and pictures in a book, or try the techniques described under 'massage' on page 163).

For more information
To obtain a list of qualified practitioners in your area contact one of the following organisations (see the 'Useful addresses' section, pages 201 and 206):

- Aromatherapy Consortium;

- International Federation of Professional Aromatherapists;

- Bookshops and most libraries carry a range of suitable books on aromatherapy or ask the organisations above for an up-to-date list of recommended books.

Bach Flower Remedies

These remedies are named after the trained medical and homeopathic doctor, Edward Bach, who researched the healing power of plants in the 1930s. He believed that the characteristics of disorders, whether physical or psychological, could be treated by a cure drawn from plants, sunlight, spring water and fresh air. In practice the Remedies tend to be used to treat psychological symptoms. This does not imply that the conditions are imagined, simply that they stem from whole body experiences that affect the mind as well as the body. Pain is a good example as, no matter what its origin is, the outcome makes people feel worried, depressed, exhausted, irritable and panicky.

People have always made use of medicinal herbs, but the thirty-eight Bach Flower Remedies claim to use the essential energy within the plant rather than actual plant material. The healing energy is stored in a preserving liquid that can be bought in a concentrated form known as the stock remedy. The concentrated forms are then diluted by mixing with pure water and an alcohol preservative. It is usual to combine several concentrates together to form the required final treatment. Because the action of Bach Remedies is mild, they cannot result in unpleasant reactions or side effects and can be used by all age groups. Although orthodox medicine cannot offer a sound reason for their claimed effects, practitioners believe that, by looking at psychological symptoms, people are encouraged to review other aspects of their behaviour, lifestyle and attitudes and this self-awareness contributes towards the healing process.

Bach Flower Remedies are available at many health shops and through specially trained therapists. They are intended primarily as a form of self-help treatment and it is therefore very easy to understand which Remedy is best for you and prepare it with the help of a book or leaflet. The following list gives suggestions about how the Remedies can be used. If you plan to treat yourself, you need to read about them in more depth:

- For exhaustion and feeling drained of energy by long-standing problems, use Olive.

- For the after-effects of accident, shock, fright and grief, use Star of Bethlehem.

- For apprehension for no known reason, use Aspen.

- For tension, fear, uncontrolled and irrational thoughts, use Cherry Plum.

Rescue Remedy
Five of the Flower Remedies – Cherry Plum, Clematis, Impatiens, Rock Rose and Star of Bethlehem – were combined by Dr Bach into an emer-

gency treatment he called 'Rescue Remedy'. It can be used for a number of problems associated with shock and injury to help create a calm, soothing feeling. It can be bought as a ready-prepared liquid, spray or cream preparations for internal or external treatment and can be used on cuts, bites or after a traumatic experience.

For more information

● To find your nearest trained practitioner and details of publications, tapes and educational material contact the Bach Centre (see page 202).

● *The Twelve Healers and Other Remedies* by Edward Bach. The CW Daniel Company Ltd.

Homeopathy

Homeopathy uses tiny amounts of natural substances to enhance the body's own healing power. The practice is centuries old and is widely used as the sole form of treatment or as a complement to orthodox medicine. The name 'homeopathy' (or 'homoeopathy') is derived from two Greek words – 'homoeos' (similar) and 'pathos' (disease). The principle is that the patient is given minute doses of a substance that, in a healthy person, would cause similar signs and symptoms to those presented by the ill person. By creating a similar condition, the homeopathic remedy stimulates the body to heal itself. The skill lies in knowing the potency of the substances and matching these to the specific signs and symptoms described by the patient. Treatments are prescribed individually. Occasionally, symptoms may worsen but this is usually a short-term effect, an early stage of the healing process.

The remedies are prepared in a unique way, by repeatedly diluting and shaking plant and mineral extracts or substances that cause sensitivity (eg house dust). Arnica is one example of a homeopathic remedy used to treat muscular back pain. Unlike herbal medicine, in which only the direct effects of plants are used, homeopathic remedies are designed to treat the whole person, not just the illness, so the person's overall physical and emotional state would be assessed. There are few diseases or conditions for which homeopathy cannot be used, although there is still the need to use orthodox medical treatments. Homeopathy cannot reverse what is irreversible and, if long term orthodox treatments have suppressed the body's natural healing powers, these may take a while to regenerate.

Practitioners are trained in homeopathic medicine and many also have a general medical qualification. Homeopathic medicine is available through the NHS but it may not be possible to find practitioners in all areas of the UK.

For more information

To find your nearest homeopathic practitioner contact:

- British Homeopathic Association (see page 203);

- Society of Homeopaths (see page 209);

- Homeopathic Medical Association (see page 205) (to find your nearest homeopathic doctor).

Massage

Therapeutic touch, particularly from Eastern cultures, has long been associated with helping to heal people who are sick and distressed. However, massage is now much more widely accepted in Western society. Unfortunately, the term 'massage' can conjure up visions of disreputable 'parlours' from the back streets of the world. Physiotherapists are trained and skilled in massage techniques which are used by sports people and as a complement to everyday medicine.

The massage described here is intended only as a method of relieving stress and discomfort that can be done by a professional therapist or performed at home. Touch is one of our earliest forms of communication, so use it as a way of helping someone else or allowing them to ease your pain. As a quick energiser, stimulator or salve for aching muscles there is no better treatment.

Simple massage is excellent for reducing acute pain and also works well on more chronic muscular tension. Massage brings pain relief by activating several body functions: it speeds up the circulation, which in turn helps to reduce swelling and promote healing; it stimulates the A-beta fibres which close the 'Gate' (see page 17); and the techniques used by masseurs create a feeling of pleasure which modifies pain perception.

Giving a basic massage requires little training and you are unlikely to do any harm because you are not interfering with body systems in an intrusive sense. It may need to be approached quite carefully, however, as some people find it difficult to touch (or be touched by) another person in a non-relationship, non-professional situation. Look upon it as a stroking action that soothes the skin and eases tense muscles. Traditional or Swedish massage uses three main actions: stroking, kneading and striking. The first two are the most useful movements for untrained people to use at home. The best places to start are the forehead, shoulders and arms. That way you can provide relief from tension without either of you feeling uncomfortable or embarrassed.

It is also easy to self-massage. If you are feeling tired or have a tension headache try applying basic forehead and neck strokes on yourself, using ready-made aromatherapy oils. Remember, essential oils must never be used neat but always in a base or carrier oil. If stiff joints and muscles make this type of movement difficult ask someone else to help.

Before you start

There are a few general rules you and the person helping you with the massage should follow if you are to gain the greatest benefit from it.

- Choose appropriate surroundings and get into comfortable positions, warm and free from external interruptions – a chair in the lounge is fine.

- Remove all relevant jewellery and make sure fingernails are short.

- Both of you need to spend a few minutes relaxing before the massage starts, because tension from the giver can be transmitted to the receiver.

- The person giving the massage needs to warm their hands and rest them on the other person for a short while, to set up contact.

- Choose a pleasant-smelling oil and put it in a warm dish nearby so that one hand can be dipped into it without changing the rhythm. Give firm, even strokes, applying pressure without hurting. Keep contact with the skin throughout, because the massage should feel like a continuous flowing movement.

- Change the pressure in different areas of the body (ie light over the bony parts and stronger over the muscle). Most people are not firm enough when they first start to massage. It is important for the person receiving the massage to give feedback, letting the other know what feels good.

- Avoid heavy pressure directly over the spine.

- The areas around the upper trunk are most prone to tension: shoulders, arms, neck and forehead.

- When the massage has finished, the person who has been massaged should spend about 20 minutes resting to maximise the feeling.

Relieving muscle tension

If you are giving a massage to someone who is particularly tense, you will feel areas of lumpy, 'knotted' muscle. Pay special attention to these taut places by kneading with your thumbs and the heels of your palms and smoothing the surrounding areas. These areas may be tender, so take care and listen to the person's reactions. All the methods below start in the same way:

1 The person receiving the massage sits in a comfortable upright chair with you standing behind. Clip or tie back long hair if necessary.

2 Warm your hands by rubbing them together and lightly coat them with a base oil, massage oil or an aromatherapy oil mixture. A massage can be done over clothing (without oil) with good effect, especially if you are not at home.

Forehead

1 Place both hands on the centre of the person's forehead, with fingertips touching, and then use firm, sweeping strokes outwards and back in a circular motion, repeating several times. Keep the movement continuous by replacing one hand with the other.

2 Move your hands in two directions: first sweep upwards towards the hairline and then downwards towards the cheekbones.

3 Finish by resting your hands for a few seconds. Ask your partner how they feel, because it is important for both of you that the massage feels right. They should feel relieved and uplifted, and you will probably feel equally soothed.

Neck and shoulders: method one

1 Place your hands on the person's neck, just below the ears, with fingers touching; in a continuous movement, sweep your hands across the shoulders and stop at the tops of the arms.

2 Repeat several times.

3 Finish by resting your hands for a few seconds. The other person should feel that tension in the neck and shoulders has been swept away.

Neck and shoulders: method two

1 Position yourself as for method one, but start with your hands at the neck end of the shoulders, palms cupped over the shoulder muscle.

2 Keeping your hands in contact with the shoulders, use the flat part of your thumbs to knead (circular pressure) the area at the back of the neck in as wide a sweep as the thumbs can reach. Do not place pressure directly over the spine.

3 Do this as long as the other person feels comfortable. (This area can become very knotty with tension and is a good place to self-massage.)

4 If the person you are giving the massage to has a tension head-ache, knead more up towards the base of the skull.

Arms

1 Prepare as before and place the person's arm on a protective towel, palm facing down.

2 Put both of your hands on the back of their lower arm and, using a firm movement, glide both hands up to the elbow.

3 Separate your hands and slide them down again, gripping round the arm, and off the end of the hand.

4 Using both hands, knead the back of the forearm, working from wrist to elbow.

5 Repeat the sequence on the upper arm.

6 Next massage the elbow with a circular movement. Use plenty of oil, because this area can be dry and becomes sore if the elbows are regularly rested in bed or on chair arms.

7 Ask the person to raise their forearm. Using your thumbs, knead the front of the forearm from wrist to elbow. Repeat several times.

8 Finish the arm massage by lightly stroking (feathering movement) from the top of the arm to the fingertips. Repeat several times and then do the other arm.

9 If someone finds a massage to the whole arm to be tiring, try massaging just the lower arms and hands.

For more information
- To obtain a list of qualified practitioners of therapeutic massage, contact the UK College for Complementary Health Care Studies (address on page 210).

Music therapy

Listening to music (a form of cognitive therapy) can be an excellent form of distraction that works on several levels. The effect of listening to music, or actually playing a musical instrument, is thought to trigger the production of endorphins and, depending on the choice of music, can be a powerful motivator to help release emotions; gentle-type music soothes and relaxes the mind, while passionate pieces can help to liberate deeper feelings. Listening to music is relatively easy, even in a crowded place; witness the number of people who can be seen wearing personal stereo earphones on public transport or even at work. The profusion of equipment and choice of methods, such as audiotapes or compact discs (CDs), mean that music therapy can be used almost anywhere. If the mechanical means are unavailable, why not hum to yourself or tap out the rhythm to a tune playing in your mind.

Reflexology

Reflexology also complements orthodox medicine, and involves massaging reflex areas in the body, found most commonly in the feet and hands, that correspond to all parts of the body. Practitioners believe that healing is encouraged by applying pressure to these points to free blockages in energy pathways. The reflex points are laid out to form a 'map' of the body, the right and left feet reflecting the right and left sides. Both feet are used to give whole body treatment and it is an ideal way to boost circulation.

The method has been used for several thousand years and is described in ancient Chinese and Egyptian writings. It does not claim to cure all problems but many conditions respond well to reflexology, especially those related to stress – such as migraine, generalised pain and digestive disorders.

Warning: The powerful effects of reflexology make it unsuitable for people with certain conditions where manipulation of the feet may not be sensible; for example, arthritis, osteoporosis and inflammation of the veins. A reflexologist takes a full history from the person and, where there is a risk of foot damage, the treatment is given with extra care or not at all, depending on the judgement of the therapist.

To start with, the practitioner will examine the feet for signs of the primary causes of conditions, which may originate from another system of the body. Then they will move on to precise massage. This involves applying firm pressure with the thumbs to all parts of the feet that correspond to the body areas giving problems. These related areas in the foot feel especially tender when massaged and the level of tenderness indicates the degree of imbalance in the body. The skill of the reflexologist lies in their ability to interpret the tenderness and apply the correct pressure, bearing in mind that some people have more sensitive feet than others. The number of treatments will vary according to the condition and the response. Reflexology is a relaxing therapy that relies on the healing power of touch rather than substances. At the end of each session people usually feel very warm and contented.

Janet is a qualified reflexologist
'When my father was dying of cancer, it was lovely to be able to massage his feet using reflexology techniques. It was a way of being close to him and communicating my love and care, even after he had lost the power to speak. And he was able to let me know it helped him.'

For more information

To find your nearest practitioner contact:

- Association of Reflexologists (see page 202)

- International Federation of Reflexologists (see page 206)

- The organisations above will provide a booklist or you can use a bookshop or library.

Reiki

Reiki is an ancient form of natural healing which originated in the Eastern countries of Tibet, India and China many centuries ago. It was rediscovered in the late nineteenth century by Dr Mikao Usui in the Sanskrit teachings from the days of the Buddha. The word Reiki is Japanese in origin. 'Rei' means 'universal' and 'ki' means 'life energy', similar to 'chi' in Chinese and 'prana' in Sanskrit. Reiki is the vital force that flows through all living things and which can be stimulated for the purpose of healing. It is thought that Reiki works at physical, mental, emotional and spiritual levels and, by balancing and strengthening these elements, activates the body's natural ability to heal itself. Reiki practitioners have been trained (attuned) up to three levels: Reiki One (level one) places an emphasis on self-healing and how to practise the techniques on another person; Reiki Two (level two) consists of further attunement which enhances the ability to amplify and channel the life force, including sending 'distant' healing to people, places and situations; Reiki Masters (level three) attunes the person to yet higher vibrational energy, which heightens their personal abilities and brings a stronger sense of self empowerment. Reiki Masters are trained to a level that enables them to teach and pass attunements to students.

For more information

- There are many sites linked to Reiki on the Internet if you like to browse online. For example, you could start with the UK Reiki Federation (see page 210) which gives information about self regulation, standards, and lists of practitioners across the country.

Visualisation

Visualisation is believed to influence the brain centres that control hormone and immune systems and helps to strengthen the healing process. Otherwise known as 'guided imagery'; it uses a method similar to meditation but needs less concentration and is easier to perform. The pictures that a person sees in their mind usually involve all five senses and can be real or a dreamlike illusion. The technique works well whether it is done alone or with someone else. Therapists use visualisation as a healing exercise to help lift the effects of chronic illness, such as anxiety and depression, and to create a positive attitude towards life-threatening illnesses. The technique can have powerful psychological effects and is often recommended as an effective form of pain relief.

Using it at home is an excellent way to shut out other stressful thoughts and to mentally take yourself on a journey or concentrate on an object that induces pleasure. The procedure works by creating a sense of contentment so that the brain responds to this lack of threat by telling the systems of the body to go into rest rather than alert mode. The reverse will happen if you visualise an unpleasant image. You may have noticed that if you think about a difficult situation, your body immediately responds by rousing itself for action, even though the event is imagined.

If your illness makes it difficult for you to travel far in real life, you can take a break from the reality that is getting you down and mentally 'visit' a place that you have enjoyed in the past without the effort of journey. First, you need to sit or lie comfortably in a quiet place and decide where you want to go, then create an imaginary 'guided' tour along familiar paths. Start and finish your journey using similar words to these: *'I am closing my eyes … Today I will visit…'*. Finish your journey by saying *'It is time to bring my visit to an end and come back home'*. Then, open your eyes, gently stretch your limbs and start to think about the present. Alternatively, you can visualise a single item such as a picture or a fantasy garden. Whatever you choose, as you practise the routine, try to bring all of your senses into play; for example, in a fantasy walk on the beach you could think about the sea, the birds, the sand and the rocks, 'images' that can be smelled, heard, seen, touched and tasted, in your mind.

Philip, who with his wife Beth, had moved away from the sea to be close to their daughter, after Beth had a stroke
'When my wife was feeling homesick and in some pain from her stiffness, to distract her I would say "let's go for a walk together along the cliff". And we would shut our eyes and walk for miles in our minds. It gave us so much pleasure we could almost smell the sea.'

Other therapies

There are many other types of therapy that can be used to complement each other and orthodox medicine. You can find out more about the therapies listed below, and others, at your local library or on the Internet:

- **Ayurvedic medicine** Practised widely in India, this all-embracing form of medicine deals with every aspect of a person's physical, mental and spiritual health, emphasising and promoting prevention alongside treatment.

- **Biofeedback** The therapist uses a machine (similar to a lie detector) to measure and monitor changes in people's physical and mental states such as body temperature and brain wave patterns. The person is then taught to control the way their body behaves using a range of calming techniques, including relaxation and visualisation.

- **Chiropractic and osteopathy** These therapies relieve pain through joint manipulation (see pages 130 and 134).

- **Herbal medicine** Herbalists use the potent healing properties of plants. Note that these preparations must always be used with caution; like all drugs, they can have unwanted (side) effects.

- **Hypnotherapy** A hypnotist will induce a trance-like state to bring about physical and mental changes and it is possible to learn self-hypnosis from a trained therapist or a book.

- **Hydrotherapy** Water treatments are used to purify and heal the body.

- **Shiatsu** This type of massage originated in Japan. It is based on the idea that good health depends on a balanced flow of energy through specific channels in the body.

- **T'ai-chi Ch'uan** (and/or **Qi Gong**) This therapy can be described as 'meditation in motion'.

For more information
The following organisations would all give you advice and supply you with further details of specialist organisations and practitioners (see the 'Useful addresses' section at the end of the book) or ask at your local library:

- British Holistic Medical Association (BHMA);

- Centre for Study of Complementary Medicine;

- Council for Complementary and Alternative Medicine;

- Depression Alliance (branches in England, Scotland and Wales);

- Institute of Complementary Medicine;

- National College of Hypnosis and Psychotherapy;

- National Federation of Spiritual Healers;

- No Panic;

- *Reader's Digest Family Guide to Alternative Medicine*, published by Reader's Digest.

- *Know Your Complementary Therapies*, by Eileen Inge Herzberg. Published by Age Concern Books.

Conclusion

Stress is normal in small amounts and harmful when it becomes so severe that it causes *distress*. The warning signs are common to everyone; however, some people because of personality type or a previous unpleasant experience react to pressure more quickly than others. The key to managing stress is learning to recognise where pressures are coming from, and then working towards changing the situation or accepting that some situations cannot be controlled.

When your body gives off the tell-tale signals that tension is rising, try to calm yourself. Slow your movements, breathe quietly and relax your muscles. Let your shoulders drop and unwind all the parts of your body that have become twisted together. Use your support systems and don't feel it is a weakness to ask for help or show signs of emotion. Crying or trembling are good ways to relieve tension, but don't try to suppress the emotion as the extra effort creates more tension. Some complementary treatments provide excellent ways of relieving tension and giving yourself a reward, as well as helping with the pain. They should always be used alongside orthodox medicine, never as substitutes for conventional treatment.

The next chapter helps you to move forward by outlining ways to achieve a healthy lifestyle.

6 Looking at your lifestyle

Although many aspects of health (such as family history), are fixed, it is never too late to make changes for the better or to make the best of your current state of health. The thought of planning lifestyle changes may be daunting, especially if chronic pain makes you feel listless and disheartened. However, none of the suggestions here involve major changes, and not all the suggested changes will apply to you, so pick out the information that is relevant. You could start by looking at your diet and exercise routine as even small changes can strengthen your body if it has been neglected in the course of the illness. For example, being overweight can aggravate some painful conditions such as arthritis of the joints. The extra weight is a burden on the joints and it also affects the ability to take regular exercise.

Other areas to think about are regulating sleep patterns, stopping smoking, adopting a sensible alcohol intake, reducing boredom and dealing with any relationship difficulties. If you feel you need help with any health-related issue, ask to speak to your practice nurse initially, who should be able to offer direct advice or point you elsewhere.

Healthy eating

Diet is an important factor in any health programme. You may have become overweight or have been neglecting to eat properly. As well as having an adverse effect on good health, either type of eating behaviour can actually be caused by ill health. So the effects can be circular.

To help break such a circle, menus can be designed to build up strength or reduce calories – or to aid a specific disorder, depending on what dietary regime is required. A review of what you eat could be one of the first steps towards feeling healthier, and modifying your diet is something that is relatively easy to do.

Some people inherit a tendency to be a certain shape, and others gain or lose weight more readily than the next person. In basic terms, anyone who eats more, or fewer, calories than they burn up will usually go up or down in weight. The simple rules for controlling weight are:

- eat foods that are energy-rich to put on weight;
- eat foods that are calorie-reduced to lose weight.

When cutting back or increasing your calories, it is important to keep an eye on the nutritional content of the diet and not reduce your intake of valuable vitamins and minerals. If you have a 'picky' appetite, select foods that give a good value per calorie.

Eating problems

People who are unwell may lose weight because they stop eating properly. If this is the case with you, check the list below to identify the reasons why you might be struggling to regain an interest in food. For example, are you:

- Too tired to eat?
- Feeling bloated and constipated?
- Suffering from indigestion after eating?
- Suffering from the side effects of medication?

Finding solutions

For general self-help and pick-me-up tips you could try the following suggestions:

- eat foods that trigger your tastebuds;
- serve smaller meals on a smaller plate to avoid the overwhelming sight of a large helping;
- try eating when you feel peckish, especially finger foods which are easy to eat;
- keep food light – eating stodgy, hard-to-chew food saps energy quickly;
- ensure food is moist as this will be easier to eat than dry food;

- lubricate a dry mouth with flavoured ice-cubes or chunks of pine-apple;

- liquidise foods into easy-to-swallow drinks using milk or fruit juice as fluid;

- keep the freezer well stocked with a choice of refreshing ice-creams;

- try all-in-one meal drinks and use these as a drink after or instead of a meal (some makes are available on prescription);

- avoid rich spicy food if this causes indigestion; conversely, if your sense of taste is reduced try 'pepping' up taste buds with strongly flavoured foods;

- use a straw if your mouth is sore or if it is easier to drink lying down;

- try a glass of sherry as an aperitif (see Alcohol, page 187);

- increase the proportion of fibre-rich/high residue foods if constipation is a problem due to the side effects of painkillers and speak to your doctor, a pharmacist or a nurse about taking gentle laxatives;

- increase the proportion of foods that bind the stools (reduced fibre/low residue foods) if diarrhoea is causing discomfort – and seek advice.

Build-up diet

This way of eating is devised to help people maintain or build up their weight. It involves introducing into the diet foods that are high in energy and protein, with the emphasis on richness and increased calories. Many people who are unwell experience eating problems and everyone needs a certain level of energy to maintain their body mass, even if they are very inactive. A diet that is advised for someone who is losing weight, or to help increase weight, is designed especially for that purpose. It is not recommended long term for people who are eating well.

Choose a selection of foods regularly from the following lists when preparing meals, to help increase calories.

- **High energy foods** Bread, pasta, cereals, cake, sweet biscuits and glucose sweets.

- **High protein foods** Meat, poultry, fish, beans, lentils, eggs, milk and cheese – but to reduce the risk of infection cook eggs well and avoid dairy products made from unpasteurised milk.

- **Rich fatty foods** Oils, butter, margarine, fatty meats and oily fish, full-fat dairy products (eg fresh cream), nuts and mayonnaise. Look for labels that state 'whole milk' and 'full-fat' rather than products that claim to be 'low-fat' or 'light'.

- **Vitamins and minerals** While vitamins and minerals are contained in most foods, some of the best sources are raw or lightly cooked fruit and vegetables with the skins intact. Ask your doctor whether taking supplements would be beneficial if your diet is restricted in any way.

If you feel frail and have lost weight, use subtle ways to introduce extra goodness without adding too much bulk. For example:

- Add extra milk or cream to soups, puddings, custard, mashed potato, breakfast cereals and drinks in the form of fortified milk foods (available from pharmacies), evaporated or condensed milk or dried milk powder. Use milk when the recipe states water.

- Add extra lentils, split peas, beans or egg noodles to meat stews and casseroles.

- Put a spoonful of real cream, rich ice-cream or condensed milk on to puddings.

- Use extra honey or syrup on breakfast cereals or porridge (made with milk or single cream).

- Keep a selection of nibbles, such as peanuts, crisps and dried fruits, in handy dishes about the house.

- Spread butter, margarine and mayonnaise more thickly, and add to mashed potato and vegetables.

Finding specialist dietary advice

It is not within the scope of this book to offer specific dietary advice for particular illnesses and disorders. However, an impressive range of material is readily available for those people who wish to investigate the field more fully. If that thought is off-putting, you can check out the research already done by many health-related charities or speak to a dietitian or nutritionist. Information can be found in the general media, in books and on the Internet. Topics to look out for cover, for example:

- Why certain diseases develop.

- Ways to boost your body's defence against general and specific disorders.

- Special diets which help to combat named diseases.

- Food groups that help to promote good health and well-being.

A note of advice: Some of the material and products you will find have been well researched and their use is promoted by mainstream, medical practitioners. Other examples may be less well examined and may make health claims that cannot be substantiated. Before embarking on a special diet that you have found for yourself, without the aid of a health professional, you are advised to consult your GP or hospital team to ensure the suitability of the programme.

For more information

- *What really works in natural health: the only guide you will ever need,* by Susan Clark, published by Bantam Press or to order by telephone call The Sunday Times Books Direct on 0870 165 8585.

- *Health Defence,* by Dr Paul Clayton, published by Accelerated Learning Systems Ltd from most bookshops.

- British Association of Nutritional Therapists (for address see page 202).

- British Society for Allergy, Environmental and Nutritional Medicine (for address see page 203).

- Institute for Optimum Nutrition (for address see page 206).

Exercise

Exercise is good news for everyone, even if you are not particularly mobile. There is rarely a reason not to exercise in some way as you can moderate the level to suit your capabilities. The information here can only be written in a general way, so before you start to take any form of exercise, you must check with your doctor first and be sure you understand what is suitable. Because pain can have so many different causes, certain types of exercise might be suitable for some people, but not for others. Indeed, in other cases they might actually be contraindicated. For example, achieving suppleness can be good for many conditions but exercise that entails weight bearing may do untold harm to fragile joints. Many people still hold the belief that exercise is likely to do them more harm than good – that the pain is there as a warning. In acute attacks that is true, but doctors now understand that 'fear avoidance' can actually slow down recovery. A current view, for example, is that specific exercises can be tremendously important in treating low back pain – but such thinking would have been extremely rare a few years ago.

Plan your exercise programme sensibly, perhaps with advice from a physiotherapist or occupational therapist at the pain clinic or local hospital, or your surgery or health centre, as they are skilled in rehabilitation after illness and will advise you about how far to extend your programme and how much pain you should endure safely. Always start gently with a mild physical activity. Perhaps ask a friend or relative to join you – a shared activity is much more pleasurable than exercising in isolation.

Lucy's story

Lucy is a former nurse who injured her back at the age of twenty, when lifting and moving patients. She was treated with physiotherapy at the time and had no further trouble for many years. However, when she was in her forties the site of this old injury became extremely sensitive and Lucy has suffered from intermittent lower back pain ever since.

Although there have been a number of occasions when acute episodes have meant Lucy needed to see a doctor, she prefers to use self-management techniques. For the past four years she has been seeing a chiropractor on a regular basis (every three months if all is well, more frequently if necessary). Lucy believes what she has to put up with is relatively minor compared to many people's problems and it has never occurred to her to ask for referral to a pain clinic.

Lucy takes over-the-counter analgesics when necessary (either paracetamol or ibuprofen). She keeps an ice pack in the fridge for acute episodes, and sometimes uses a 'deep heat' spray or a cream containing aloe vera and eucalyptus oil to provide local relief. She enjoys walking and swimming, and has been given a number of specific exercises by her chiropractor which she is encouraged to do at least once a day. She says 'I know I should do them, and they do help. It's just not always easy to motivate myself last thing at night when I'm tired. But I am always woken up early in the morning by pain and stiffness in my lower back if I don't do them'.

The advantages of exercise are well proven as a way of increasing physical strength, mobility and mental well-being. It's also very good for reducing stress as it boosts the hormones that produce feelings of happiness and the movement gently relaxes muscle tension. Muscles work more smoothly, with less effort, if they are made to work regularly. The Health Development Agency recommends exercise that boosts the three S's – strength, suppleness and stamina – all within moderation. Ask at your surgery or health centre whether there are any health-linked initiatives being run in conjunction with your local sports centre. Many doctors recognise the health benefits and encourage this type of supported scheme.

Exercising safely

Whichever activity you choose, it is important to be aware of a few safety rules, even after you have been given approval to get going:

- Start exercising gradually and build up exertion levels at a rate that feels comfortable. No-one should behave as if they are training for the Olympics.

- Don't exercise for at least two hours after a meal as the digestive system places an automatic demand on the blood supply to digest the food.

- Wear clothes that are loose and comfortable and shoes or trainers that provide adequate support.

- Never rush straight into the most strenuous part of the activity. Start and stop at a gentle pace to allow muscles to warm up and cool down before and after exercise.

- Drink plenty of fluids, but not alcohol as this increases dehydration.

- Stop immediately if there are any signs of breathlessness, chest pains or feeling unwell in any way. If exercise causes problems, however minor, it would be wise to inform the doctor before continuing with the programme.

Ringing the changes

The following activities are classed as leisure hobbies rather than exercises for fitness fanatics; some can be done alone, some need a partner. If you would like to join a club, look in the local *Yellow Pages* or ask for details at the library.

- **Walking** This is a good choice if you have been inactive as it boosts stamina and allows fitness to build up at a steady rate. Walking needs no special equipment, it is free, relaxing, and pleasurable to share with a companion. Start with short walks and increase the pace and distance over a few weeks. Remember to wear comfortable shoes.

- **Swimming** Another good exercise for people of all ages, swimming combines the three S's – stamina, strength and suppleness. It is often described as the ideal activity and can be a great stress reducer. Swimming is especially good for people who are overweight or have joint or back problems as the water supports the body. Most people live within reasonable distance of a swimming pool and the charges are often reduced for certain categories of people. Look out for sessions especially reserved for people with disabilities.

- **Cycling** This is another good exercise for improving on the three S's. It is recommended for people who are overweight and helps reduce stress as well as being pleasurable. Cycling in the fresh air is the best choice but an indoor cycle machine provides an alternative way to 'get pedalling'.

- **Golf** Golf is a great energiser. It helps build up stamina and strength, and provides fresh air and an opportunity to make new friends. Start off gently with a few holes and stop to enjoy the scenery.

- **Gardening** (See page 183)

- **Bowling** Join a club to get the best advantage from indoor and grass bowls and try the ten pin variety with younger family members for some challenging play. All forms of bowling are excellent for suppleness and relaxation.

- **Badminton** This enjoyable game suits all ages as long as partners of similar ability are matched. At club level it can be quite a vigorous sport, so don't get drawn into competitive games until you have built up skills at a pace that is comfortable. Check with your doctor before starting this type of exercise.

- **Exercise and dance classes** These are readily available in most areas. Ask at a leisure centre about classes to suit your age and ability level. Both types of exercise are good for stamina, strength and suppleness. Tea dances are especially relaxing and enjoyable.

- **Yoga** Good for suppleness and strengthening body muscles, yoga is an excellent form of exercise. It will help you to control movements and breathing, and will encourage muscle relaxation.

- **Home-based exercise** If getting out and about is a problem, ask to speak to a physiotherapist or occupational therapist (or see EXTEND below) about the range of activities that can be practised at home. For example, movement and exercise (perhaps accompanied by music or a video) is possible even for people whose mobility is limited or who are chairbound.

Leg cramps

Even small increases in exertion may cause leg cramps for some people, particularly if they take up exercising after a long period of inactivity. Your doctor will advise about taking exercise if leg cramps are painful (see also page 72).

For more information
- For details of local adult sport and leisure activity classes contact your local education authority, community centre, or private leisure centres.

- The Sports Council provides general information about all sports (see page 209).

- EXTEND provides recreational movement to music for older and less able people. EXTEND is active in many parts of the UK and trained teachers provide one-to-one sessions for those who require specialised exercise (see page 205).

Gardening

For non-gardening addicts, take note that this activity is a wonderfully relaxing way to combine exercise with fresh air and do lots of bending and stretching. Recent research into horticultural therapy has shown it to be very beneficial for people who are depressed. However, for many people what started as a hobby may well have developed into a life-long 'passion'. But what if you have a bad back or no longer have the physical strength to garden in the way you have become accustomed over many years? The inability to continue doing something you love is bound to cause distress. The extent to which you can carry on garden-ing will clearly be dictated by your particular disability, and here a medical professional must advise you about personal levels of ability and safety. Perhaps this is one of the many areas that you will have to settle for a compromise. Fortunately, for most people there will be some method of gardening that helps to fill the gap; for example, you could try:

- Raising the level of the flower/vegetable beds to avoid the need to bend over.

- Exploring the huge range of tools that are available to aid disabled people.

- Setting yourself realistic goals and putting your 'pacing' techniques into practice.

- Finding a gardening 'partner' or 'buddy' among family or friends who will share the tasks with you.

- Joining a gardening club or checking out a nearby allotment scheme so that you can discuss gardening matters and pass on your expertise to newer, less experienced members and suggest a 'buddy' scheme that is run through the club.

- Downsizing to gardening in pots on a patio or the kitchen table – it may feel like a window box approach if you have been used to large-scale gardening but it still involves getting close to live plants.

- Visiting country/town houses with gardens that are open to the public and parks and annual garden shows where you can touch and smell the plants.

- Continuing to thumb through your gardening books and cata-logues because even second-hand browsing can bring pleasure and is a form of 'visualisation'.

A better night's sleep

Pain and tension are at the heart of many sleep problems, when bodies ache and thoughts race around the brain. If pain is making you sleep badly there are things that you can do to complement your medication; for example by practising the relaxation techniques described in Chapter 5. You also need to be aware that older people naturally take longer to fall asleep, are more likely to wake during the night and tend to wake earlier in the morning. Sharing a bed with someone who is restless due to night pain can have considerable effects on carers.

Dorothy cares for her husband, who has kidney failure
'He gets a lot of bone pain and restless legs, especially at night. Sometimes, the only way I can sleep is to go into the spare room. But I always hate having to do that because it feels like I'm abandoning him.'

Tips to help settle at night

The following suggestions may be helpful:

- Go to bed at a regular time, with a regular routine.
- Make everything as cosy as possible, with a warm room and a comfortable bed.
- Don't eat a rich, heavy meal late in the day.
- Avoid stimulating drinks that contain alcohol or caffeine later in the day and choose a milky drink at bedtime.
- Cut back on evening fluids if a full bladder is the cause of waking.
- Read or listen to the radio until you naturally feel sleepy.
- If waking in the night is a problem, do something to break the rest-less mood – rather than lie tossing and turning, get up and watch some television and repeat the milky drink with a biscuit.

- Take regular exercise, but not too late in the day as strenuous exercise releases hormones that are stimulating.

- Rest and cat-nap during the day, but resist having too long a sleep as this simply reduces the amount you need at night. A 'power' nap of no more than ten minutes can be very rejuvenating.

Dealing with extreme tiredness

Fatigue is more than just being 'tired', it is feeling completely exhausted most of the time. Extreme tiredness is a problem that many ill people experience at some stage. Symptoms of fatigue may interfere with the most basic activities such as climbing stairs, brushing teeth and eating food. Shortness of breath is common and people with severe tiredness find it too arduous to carry on a conversation, concentrate to read or even watch the television. Fatigue is made worse by a combination of factors related to illness and treatments, for example, poor appetite, lack of sleep, anxiety and anaemia all contribute to the weariness caused by the pain. Trying to battle against fatigue like this increases debility, so for a while it may be easier to give in and let others take over the major tasks of shopping, laundry and household chores. Plan your day so that you can achieve the things that are most important to you, with lots of rest periods in between.

Boosting mood

People suffering from pain, particularly chronic pain, are often prone to depression and anxiety. Sometimes, coping with the pain itself can prevent people from noticing that they are actually very depressed. In such a situation, they may not connect poor appetite, poor sleep, a reduction in libido, and lack of interest in things they would normally enjoy, as part of their pain 'syndrome'.

Mavis's story
Mavis has been hurting with tension in her neck and shoulders for two and a half years. She feels the pain in her head and when it is at its worst she gets very depressed. When these bouts occur she is not interested in going out, doing any shopping or preparing meals. Mavis usually finds that going to bed helps her to get away from the pain as, fortunately, it does not keep her awake.

On a good day, when the pain is lighter, Mavis manages to do some gardening, which she really enjoys. She has also managed to continue to play bowls throughout the years she has experienced pain but at times it has been hard.

For, Mavis the three key sentiments that spring to mind in relation to her illness are 'fed up', 'depressed' and 'life not worth living'.

Mavis does believe that her husband is affected because it stops him going out if she feels down. He also has to help out a bit more around the house!

The treatment(s) that have worked best for Mavis over the years have been a combination of medication and therapies from the following lists:

Prescribed by the general practitioner or hospital consultant
* *Anti-depressants – dosulepin (dothiepin) is taken each night, also citalopram, which helps with the panic disorder.*
* *Physiotherapy, which Mavis believes has helped her the most.*

Self-help treatments
* *Aromatherapy.*

Complementary therapies
* *Osteopathy*
* *Head massage.*

Mavis has visited a pain clinic once and had an injection in the shoulder but it did not help. She had not yet attended the follow up appointment when offering to provide her story for the book.

Depression is a common symptom of chronic pain but it should never be thought of as 'normal' or an inevitable consequence of feeling pain. If you feel that you are experiencing the symptoms of depression or anxiety, no matter what level, it is possible to find a treatment that brings relief. Always tell someone from the medical team about low moods and talk over the benefits of trying out some of the following options, depending on the extent of the problem:

* being prescribed a conventional drug treatment;

* taking a herbal drug treatment (eg St John's wort);

- being referred to a psychiatric specialist (initially this could be a Registered Mental Nurse, who works in hospital and community settings);

- receiving counselling from a trained counsellor;

- contacting a helpline or self-help group or drawing on personal support networks;

- trying light therapy if mood swings are more pronounced in winter;

- practising one or more of the complementary therapies described in the previous chapter;

- finding some way of relieving boredom if that is a problem, such as a reviving or starting a new hobby, doing some volunteering or joining a group such as the University of the Third Age (see address on page 210);

- Planning a short break or a holiday (see page 196).

Periods of anxiety or depression do pass, despite the debilitating feeling at the time. One of the main sources of inner strength is feeling that your have a degree of control over the situation, so helping yourself and working with your medical team are positive steps that can boost mood and confidence.

For more information
- *Caring for someone with depression,* by Toni Battison (2004). Age Concern Books.

Alcohol

In general, the main message from doctors and scientists suggests that, for the majority of people, alcohol taken in small amounts may be beneficial and does no obvious harm. It is also acknowledged that for a small proportion of the population, alcohol can have unpleasant effects and studies have made links between alcohol and feeling low. It is unclear which comes first, however. Do bouts of heavy drinking cause people to feel depressed, or do people who are dejected turn to alcohol? Enduring chronic pain makes many people feel low in mood but not everyone is affected so directly that they turn to alcohol; it seems likely that those depressed people who over-use alcohol have an initial predisposition to depression. They may then start to drink excessively for several reasons. Alcohol has the ability to release the self-discipline that controls inhibition, and this feeling of 'letting go' might encourage depressed people to drink too much in the mistaken belief that it will relieve their mood, as in the expression 'drowning your sorrows'. They may find the effect of alcohol helps to deaden their pain, and may over-use it to that end. Some people also believe that alcohol gives courage and the energy to cope with life. Unfortunately, any relief given by alcohol soon wears off. The low feeling then appears worse, and the inclination is likely to be to increase alcohol consumption. Doctors have reported that, when questioned about alcohol intake, depressed people tend to under-estimate their drinking habits by as much as 50 per cent. In general, excessive drinking is strongly linked to many causes of illness and death including cancer, liver disease, strokes and accidental death.

In the face of evidence from many studies around the world, the most sensible advice is that alcohol should be drunk in moderation only. For the general population who are not suffering from ill health, the recommended weekly amount is a maximum of twenty standard drinks ('units') for men. Women, who are less able to metabolise alcohol because they have a smaller liver, are advised to drink no more than fourteen standard units. Everyone is advised to restrict their drinking by having at least two or even three alcohol-free days each week to give their bodies a rest. It is also important to be aware that alcoholic drinks vary in potency, and that drinks poured at home tend to be larger than standard pub measures (ie more than one 'unit' per glass).

For people suffering from ill health, the advice leans much more towards exercising caution and it is usually recommended that people taking many types of medication avoid alcohol completely, as it frequently affects the drug action. However, each patient should be assessed individually.

If you enjoy the occasional drink, check with your doctor that alcohol will have no adverse effects on your particular illness or interact with painkilling and other drugs. If permission is given, aim to stay well below the recommended levels for the general population. Some tips to help you drink safely, include:

• avoid the temptation of using alcohol as a mood booster;

• read the instruction leaflet that accompanies most tablets to check out any warning signs about adverse reactions connected

to alcohol. Symptoms might include nausea, headaches and dizziness. Study the wording carefully because in some cases it may
expressly caution people not to take alcohol with a particular drug
as the combination would be harmful; in other cases the language
may advise against anything other than occasional or minimal use
of the two substances together because, although not seriously
harmful, the reaction could be unpleasant;

- sip drinks slowly to make each glass last longer;

- avoid undiluted spirits or drinking on an empty stomach;

- try non-alcoholic wines or beers, and explore the wide range of
  soft drinks now available;

- get some help from an alcohol agency if the situation is becoming
  a problem.

For more information

- Alcohol Concern, tel: 020 7928 7377, offers information in the
  form of factsheets, leaflets and a journal but not direct advice (see
  page 201).

- Drinkline: national alcohol helpline, tel: 020 7332 0202, providing
  confidential information, help and advice about drinking to anyone, including people worried about someone else's drinking (see
  page 205).

Smoking

It is a myth that smoking may not be harmful. The facts about smoking-
related illnesses are clear. The proven evidence from a large number of
scientific studies shows that all forms of smoking (cigarettes, cigars and
pipes) damage health. Smoking is the biggest avoidable cause of premature death and ill health; the earlier a person starts to smoke the greater
their likelihood of developing smoking-related diseases. However, it is
never too late to feel the benefits of giving up, and it is one of the most
effective changes that anyone can make to improve their health.

Tobacco smoke contains many poisonous chemicals that play a significant part in the build-up of atherosclerosis, the process that 'hardens'
and 'furs up' the artery walls, and is a major cause of angina. Smoking
causes vasoconstriction thus reducing oxygen available to tissues. This

can worsen painful conditions such as angina or leg cramps (see pages 44 and 72). Moreover, chemical action makes the blood thicker, increasing the chance of blood clots. The most serious damage is caused by three main substances:

- **Carbon monoxide** This takes the place of some of the oxygen in the bloodstream, so vital organs are deprived of essential oxygen. Carbon monoxide also aggravates arterial disease, contributing to high blood pressure.

- **Tar** This lines the tissues of the lungs, reducing the amount of oxygen getting across to the bloodstream. Tar also causes irritation and inflammation of the lungs, leading to the development of chronic bronchitis and emphysema, two conditions that can eventually contribute to heart failure. (Of course, there is also the risk of developing lung cancer.)

- **Nicotine** This is an addictive substance that acts as a mental depressant but its chief danger is its ability to act swiftly on artery walls, causing them to contract very strongly. These muscle spasms vastly reduce the flow of blood to the heart muscle and are the major cause of angina.

Most people do understand that smoking is bad for their health, especially if a family member has developed a tobacco-related disease, principally illnesses that affect the respiratory and circulatory systems. For example, painful leg cramps can become worse in people who smoke regularly and chronic bronchitis and emphysema are common and often fatal illnesses resulting from years of using tobacco products.

If you smoke, you may have been advised to give up. But the problem often lies, not in the acceptance that cigarette smoke is the culprit, but in the ability to actually stop. Quitting smoking is not an easy thing to do as long-term smokers are usually addicted to nicotine and may suffer severe withdrawal symptoms. It can be particularly difficult during a bout of illness when stress levels are increased by pain and you feel anxious about the future. If your desire to smoke is very strong, attempting to give up while you are feeling low may not be realistic. Be ready to take positive steps when you are over the worst of the illness or when the effects of the smoke and tobacco chemicals are giving serious symptoms. Learning to relax, or using other techniques described in Chapter Five, all help to take the mind off the unpleasant withdrawal symptoms that most people experience when they cut back or stop smoking abruptly. Be prepared to draw on all your reserves of willpower and make use of a number of tips listed below.

Tips for stopping smoking

- However irritable you become, resist the temptation to start smoking again.

- Change routines so that old habits don't make it easy to light up. Identify times and places that make you feel particularly vulnerable to lighting up, and alter behaviour if necessary. For example, sit in a different chair, drink tea instead of coffee and change routines after a meal – as all of these activities may be associated with a previous smoking habit.

- Drink plenty of water, as ex-smokers need to flush the chemicals well out of their system. Fruit juice is also particularly good as vitamin C helps to rid the body of nicotine.

- Try different forms of entertainment to help combat boredom, particularly activities which involve using the hands.

- Some people like plenty of praise and support whereas other, more sensitive, people may prefer not to be reminded. Tell your friends and relatives which approach would work best for you.

- Suggest that someone tells friends and colleagues that you are giving up for health reasons. That way people are less likely to smoke in your presence and, hopefully, won't tease you for your efforts.

- Read more about the benefits of giving up. For example, after a few days your sense of taste and smell begins to return; after a few weeks your lungs are cleaner and breathing becomes easier thus improving your ability to climb stairs and cope with sudden exertion; the number and severity of angina attacks improves; and after a year the risk of a heart attack is reduced by 50 per cent.

- Add up the money that is being saved, and think of ways you can use it to treat yourself!

Smoking cannabis

Tobacco is not the only substance that can be smoked, although others such as cannabis are not legal in the UK under present law. While there have been recent arguments for the use of cannabis in the treatment of certain diseases (see page 127), its use should be restricted to strictly controlled medical situations.

For more information
* Talk to other ex-smokers or telephone the freephone helpline run by the independent charity Quitline (0800 002 200) which provides confidential and practical advice for people wanting to give up smoking.

* NHS Smoking Helpline (0800 169 0 169) offers similar help and support to give up all forms of smoking.

Sexual relationships

Sexual pleasure and painful physical conditions don't always go well together. When to resume sexual relationships after an illness or surgery, or how great the risks are for someone who has angina, are questions that many people avoid asking because of embarrassment. General advice only is offered here; specific guidance will depend very much on your personal circumstances. Your doctor will be able to reassure you about your condition, and will not be embarrassed to discuss the matter.

Generally, the advice to people with a heart conditions is to treat sex like any other type of exercise. Regular sexual activity that induces slight breathlessness is good news: it aids recovery by strengthening the heart muscle, relieves stress and adds to the feeling of well-being. Normal sex with a known partner puts a strain on the heart equivalent to climbing two flights of stairs! In the rare cases where sexual activity has brought on a heart attack there are usually other factors that contributed to the situation. A heavy meal or too much alcohol, and the excitement of having sex with a new partner or unknown person, can all put additional strain on the heart. Like any other form of exercise, it is wise to take note of how the body feels: if sexual activity causes discomfort or chest pains, stop immediately and talk to the doctor about the problem.

The key piece of advice for people with disorders affecting joints, bones and muscles or nerve pathways is likely to be – behave according to how you feel. It is unlikely that any normal type of sexual activity will harm your body; however, vigorous sexual practice may be uncomfortable or more difficult. The section below offers you some alternative and very pleasurable ways to enjoy sexual experiences.

Other ways to achieving sexual pleasure

People who have known each other and/or lived together for a period of time often become very close when one partner is ill, offering each other tremendous support through the bad moments and sharing joy and relief when times are good. People can express love for each other in many ways and the role of a carer as well as a partner is one clear example. But, however close you are to your partner, making the adjustment from a caring relationship back (or forward) into a sexual relationship, depending on levels of pain, may be a major step. It is usual for sexual interest to diminish during a period of illness, or when acute or chronic pain is a problem, and certain types of medication often accentuate lack of desire. The most common problems are:

- lowered arousal;
- reduced performance;
- feeling less pleasure;
- inability to reach orgasm;
- difficulty in achieving or maintaining an erection in men;
- premature ejaculation or difficulty ejaculating in men.

If sexual relationships have suffered between you and your partner, and you wish to continue to be sexually active, there are many ways that pleasure can be achieved other than by direct sexual intercourse. For example, kissing and caressing someone gently is a non-threatening way to give and receive comfort. Be guided by your partner's mood and be careful about expressing negative feelings. A person who is struggling to cope with their own fragile emotions may not be able to handle yours as well. Be flexible about the time of day that you explore sexual pleasure – night time, after a tiring day, may not be best time to choose. If problems persist after a reasonable time period, ask for advice from your GP or hospital clinic team. They will either be able to advise you or help you to get more specialist advice if this would be useful. The doctors who work at family planning clinics specialise in sexual health, for example, and are trained to deal with people in an older age group as well as people of child-bearing age. They would be able to reassure you both, and could recommend useful books that focus on the needs of people who are not as physically fit as they used to be.

Impotence

Peripheral vascular disease (see page 72), the condition that causes painful leg cramps, can also affect sexual performance in some men, leading to difficulty achieving or maintaining an erection. Poor blood supply to the penis may be a factor, but other causes – stress, tiredness, side effects from drugs and leaking veins that cannot retain blood in the penis – all affect the quality of an erection. If impotence is a problem for you, do seek help from a doctor because special drug treatments are available – for example, Viagra (sildenefil) and testosterone. One question that will be asked is whether there is a morning erection, as this information will help the doctor to decide whether there are physical causes. A change in drug treatment or some relaxation therapy may be all that is needed to improve the situation.

For more information

- The charity The Outsiders has a comprehensive website offering advice and information to disabled people (see page 208).

- *Intimate Relations: Living and loving in later life,* by Dr Sarah Brewer (2004). Age Concern Books (see page 216 for details of how to order; or available from most bookshops).

Transport and mobility

As you gain more control over your pain you may want to reclaim a bit of your life and venture further from home, perhaps for a shopping trip or to visit friends. If driving is restricted travel may be a problem. Look out for transport schemes for older and disabled people, available in most areas and run by local authorities and voluntary organisations. People who qualify may be able to claim back their fares to hospital.

The main schemes to help people with transport are listed below (for contact details, see Useful addresses, pages 201–210):

- **Dial-a-Ride and Community Transport Schemes** These provide door-to-door services for shopping or similar outings for people who cannot use public transport.

- **Hospital Car Schemes (also called Medical Patient Transport Schemes)** Such schemes are usually run by the ambulance service and arranged through GPs' surgeries. They are available only for people who have a medical condition and cannot get to the hospital independently. One companion is usually allowed.

- **The Blue Badge Scheme** This provides a national arrangement of parking concessions for people with severe walking difficulties who travel as drivers or passengers. Badge holders are exempted from certain parking restrictions – including free parking at on-street parking meters and for up to three hours on single and double yellow lines in England and Wales. Badges are issued for a three-year period through social services departments. Check local rules carefully, wherever you park, especially as some London Boroughs do not offer free parking arrangements. The Blue Badge can also be used in some European Union (EU) countries. Travel agents may be able to advise you or the local Tourist Information Office in the area where you are staying.

- **Motability** This charity was set up to help those disabled people who want to spend the mobility component of their Disability Living Allowance or War Pensioner's Mobility Supplement on a car or wheelchair. Vehicles may be purchased or leased and help may be available with the cost of special adaptations. A relative, friend or carer may apply and drive on behalf of a disabled person.

- **Concessionary rail fares** Most train operators have a railcard that offers concessionary fares to disabled people, giving up to one-third off a range of rail tickets. An annual charge is made for this concession. A discount may also be available to the person who accompanies you. An application form and booklet called *Rail Travel for Disabled Passengers* can be found at most stations or from the Disabled Persons Railcard Office (see page 205). All rail operators give extra help to older or disabled travellers, particularly if they have advance notice.

- **Shopmobility** Shopmobility schemes provide free wheelchair or scooter loan services in many town centres for anyone with a mobility problem. Users can usually park free or be met at the bus station or taxi rank by prior arrangement. An escort service is often available for people who are visually impaired or wheelchair users. Ask at your local town hall or see the website address for the National Federation of Shopmobility UK on page 207.

- **Taxicard** This and other similar services provide subsidised taxi fares. They are run by many local authorities for permanently disabled people who are unable to use public transport. One passenger may accompany the cardholder. Ask at your town hall.

- **Tripscope** This organisation offers a free nationwide travel and transport information and advice service for older and disabled people. Tripscope will help with planning a journey, but it is not a travel agency so cannot make bookings (see page 209).

- **The Community Transport Association** This association has services to benefit providers of transport for people with mobility problems (see page 203).

- **The Disability Living Allowance Unit** Part of the Department for Work and Pensions, this unit gives information about exemption from road tax for vehicles used exclusively by or for disabled people receiving the higher rate of the mobility component of Disability Living Allowance (DLA) or War Pensioners' Mobility Supplement. You may claim on behalf of the person you look after by completing an application form from the Benefits Agency (see page 204).

For more information

- Age Concern Factsheet 26: *Travel information for older people.*

- Contact your local authority for more information about local schemes to help with transport.

Holidays

Once you are feeling better you may benefit from a holiday, perhaps by starting off with a mini-break to build up your confidence. Your GP, practice nurse or pain clinic will be able to advise you about when the time is right, and explain the main aspects of your personal health care that you need to consider if you wish to go abroad. If you need additional advice, specialist holiday health care clinics usually offer very up-to-date information. Your surgery or health centre should be able to tell where the nearest clinic is situated. At the planning stage it would be wise to find out about the following points in case you need to make special travel arrangements or choose your destination carefully. For example, some airlines refuse to carry passengers who are still recuperating after a serious operation or accident as air turbulence during the flight or a bumpy landing may have a disabling affect. Think about the following:

- Taking certain drugs, such as strong painkillers, out of the country through customs. To avoid any difficulties at checkpoints ensure that your prescription drugs are clearly marked with your name on a proper label supplied by the pharmacist.

- Taking syringes or other equipment through the X-ray systems at airports. It may be acceptable to put some items into your non-cabin luggage, but if any piece of equipment is necessary during your journey and likely to be questioned at customs (or lost in transit), do not wait until you get to the check-in desk to ask permission to carry sharp articles in you hand luggage. You may be refused and you will certainly hold up the queue. Ask the airline or specialist holiday medical clinic in advance for guidance.

- Insurance cover may be affected if you have an existing illness. Most companies need to know in advance if this applies, and failing to inform them may invalidate your policy.

- The possible effects of heat and sunlight – both on you yourself, and on any drugs that might be affected. If this is likely to be a problem in your case, it might be advisable to look at one of the many attractive holiday destinations with a cooler climate.

- How you will cope with immobility. For example, remember to book a wheelchair at the airport and additional assistance if family members cannot manage you and the luggage; plan for regular stops if you are travelling by car, so that you can stretch aching joints; and if you are choosing to travel by coach speak to the tour company well in advance to check out their itinerary and number of comfort stops. If you are booking an aeroplane or coach seat, you need to book early if you would like to reserve a seat close to the on-board lavatory.

- Ask your doctor before booking a holiday about the danger of deep-vein thrombosis or conditions created by changes in air pressure in case your risk level is greater than the general population. It would be very upsetting (as well as costly) if the doctor advised against a certain type of holiday which you had already booked.

Holiday planning services that specifically deal with information for older or disabled people can be used, and this may reduce much of the load on you. The organisations listed below are selected from the many that provide help.

For more information

- Across Trust provides accompanied holidays and pilgrimages for sick and disabled people by means of a jumbo-ambulance. Individual or group applications are welcome (see page 201).

- Age Concern Factsheet 4: *Holidays for older people.*

- Air Transport Users Council publishes a booklet *Care in the Air* for disabled passengers (see page 201).

- RADAR (Royal Association for Disability and Rehabilitation) provides information about many aspects of disability, including accessible destinations for holidays (see page 209).

- The website www.everybody.co.uk provides information on services offered to people with disabilities by fifty major airlines. It also lists hotels in the UK that are easily accessible.

- Winged Fellowship provides respite care and holidays for physically disabled people, with or without a partner, in purpose built holiday centres and on overseas and touring holidays. Trained staff and volunteers provide care (see page 210).

Maintaining the good times

When a pain management programme has been established there are still a few things you can do to build on all your hard work and help to prevent a backward step.

- Continue taking the medication for as long as the doctor recommends. Stopping early is not a good move even if the symptoms are no longer noticeable and you feel recovered.

- Continue to visit the therapist if a 'talking' therapy has been part of the treatment programme. The frequency of the appointments can be scaled down.

- Continue any exercise routines and techniques that have been useful. This can be likened to playing a musical instrument where failure to practise soon leads to reduced skills.

- Build on the emotional strengths that have been gained. You may now have a better insight into how you think and feel, so use this self-knowledge to your advantage. At the first signs of impending stress, step up the self-help techniques before it takes a hold.

- Keep fit and active. Stimulation of both the mind and the body is a great way to help keep well at any age.

- Join a support network or self-help group for specific disorders, if one is available locally, to meet and share experiences with people in a similar state to you. If a local group does not exist (and you feel able) you could consider starting a new branch or you may prefer to receive support and newsletters long-distance; either way you can contact the appropriate national office for advice. (See list of useful addresses on pages 201–210)

- Above all don't get worried by the odd day when you find you are feeling less well. It is absolutely normal for pain levels to fluctuate, and this is not a signal that should necessarily alarm you.

John's story

The body has such a tremendous ability to heal itself! In the first few weeks after John's accident, which left him with multiple fractures, he was in a dreadful state: highly dependent on other people, knocked out and nauseated by strong painkillers which, despite maximum doses, never quite cleared the background pain, and mentally shocked. He found he was continually reliving the accident and the hours in the Accident and Emergency Department at the local hospital. He felt too exhausted even to open a newspaper. But, amazingly, just a few weeks later he was a different person, thrilled and encouraged by his own steady rate of progress.

A great many factors contributed to John's recovery: plenty of rest, mugs of milky drinks to pile in the protein and fuel the repair process, very positive support from his GP, excellent care from his physiotherapist, an understanding that high doses of painkilling drugs were necessary in the short term and an unshaking self-belief that he would be soon be back to normal.

The holistic bio/psycho/social approach to getting better worked wonders for John. Three months later he felt like a new person – two stones lighter and physically and mentally well on the path to recovery.

Conclusion

This chapter has encouraged you to focus on some of the changes that are happening to you, and has offered some hints as to how you might move forward. Adjusting to new situations is never easy, especially if the event that triggered the change was both distressing and beyond your control. We all deal with problems more effectively if we feel that an element of choice is involved and we are able to exercise some direction over the situation. With any illness it may feel that this is not the case. However, there are lots of ways that self-help can be practised and it is important to maintain a positive outlook. After a while unpleasant memories do fade, and you will be able to look ahead with greater confidence and perhaps benefit from changes in lifestyle. Whatever the long-term future holds, you will be able to access services if you need more care.

Useful addresses

Across Trust
Bridge House
70-72 Bridge Road
East Molesey
Surrey KT8 9HF
Tel: 020 8783 1355
Web: www.across.org
Provides accompanied holidays for sick and disabled people.

Action Asthma Patient Service
Freepost DR83
Ashford
Kent TN24 0YX
Tel: 020 8990 3011
Provides information for asthma sufferers.

Action for ME
PO Box 1302
Wells
Somerset BA5 1YE
Tel: 01749 670799
Web: www.afme.org.uk
Campaigns to improve the lives of people with ME.

Action on Pain
20 Necton Road
Little Dunham
Norfolk PE32 2DN
Helpline: 0845 603 1593
(9.00am-5.00pm, Monday to Friday)
Web: www.action-on-pain.co.uk
Provides support and advice to people affected by chronic pain.

Advice UK (formerly the Federation of Independent Advice Centres)
12th Floor, New London Bridge House
25 London Bridge Street
London SE1 9ST
Tel: 020 7407 4070
Web: www.adviceuk.org.uk
Promotes the provision of independent advice centres in the UK.

Age Concern England
1268 London Road
London SW16 4ER
Tel: 020 8765 7200
Web: www.ageconcern.org.uk
See page 214.

Alcohol Concern
Waterbridge House
32-36 Loman Street
London SE1 0EE
Tel: 020 7928 7377
Web: www.alcoholconcern.org.uk
Aims to raise awareness of the risk of alcohol abuse and educate people about safer drinking habits and improve existing services. Provides information only, not direct advice.

Air Transport Users Council
5th Floor, Kingsway House
103 Kingsway
London WC2B 6QX
Tel: 020 7242 3882
Web: www.caa.co.uk
Publishes a booklet, Flight Plan, which has a section for disabled passengers.

Aromatherapy Consortium
PO Box 6522
Desborough
Kettering
Northants NN14 2YX
Tel: 0870 774 3477
(10.00am-2.00pm, Monday to Friday)
Web: www.aocuk.net
For a list of qualified practitioners in your area.

Arthritic Association
One Upper Gardens
Eastbourne
East Sussex BN21 2AA
Helpline: 0800 652 3188
(10.00am-1.00pm and 2.00-4.00pm Monday to Friday)
Web: www.arthriticassociation.org.uk
Offers a natural, drug-free treatment for arthritis based on dietary guidance and herbal preparations.

Arthritis Care
18 Stephenson Way
London NW1 2HD
Tel: 020 7916 1500
Web: www.arthritiscare.
org.uk
*Provides information
and support for people
affected by arthritis.*

**Association of Charity
Officers (incorporating
the Occupational
Benevolent Funds
Alliance)**
Unicorn House
Station Close
Potters Bar
Hertfordshire EN6 3JW
Tel: 01707 651777
Web: www.aco.uk.net
*Provides information about
charities that make grants
to individuals in need.*

**Association of
Nutritional Therapists**
27 Old Gloucester Street
London WC1N 3XX
*For a list of registered
members send £2.00 plus
a large (A4) SAE.*

**Association of
Reflexologists**
27 Old Gloucester Street
London WC1N 3XX
Tel: 0870 567 3320
Web: www.aor.org.uk
*For names of
reflexologists.*

Bach Centre
Mount Vernon Ltd
Bakers Lane
Sotwell
Wallingford
Oxfordshire OX10 0PX
Tel: 01491 834678
Web: www.bachcentre.
com
*For a list of trained
practitioners and details
of publications, tapes and
educational material.*

**British Acupuncture
Council**
63 Jeddo Road
London W12 9HQ
Tel: 020 8735 0400
Web: www.acupuncture.
org.uk
*A free list of practitioners is
available by telephone or
from the website.*

**British Association
for Counselling and
Psychotherapy (BACP)**
1 Regent Place
Rugby
Warwickshire CV21 2PJ
Helpline: 0870 443 5252
Web: www.bacp.co.uk
*Publishes a directory
of counsellors and
psychotherapists in the
UK.*

**British Association of
Nutritional Therapists
(BANT)**
27 Old Gloucester Street
London WC1N 3XX
Tel: 0870 6061 1284
Web: www.bant.org.uk
*Holds a list of registered
nutritional therapists
throughout the UK.*

**British Cardiac Patients
Association**
2 Station Road
Swavesey
Cambridge CB4 5QJ
Helpline: 0800 479 2800
Web: www.bcpa.co.uk
*Offers help and advice to
cardiac patients and their
families. Has autonomous
support groups around the
country.*

**British Complementary
Medicine Association
(BCMA)**
249 Fosse Road South
Leicester LE3 1AE
Tel: 0116 282 5511
Web: www.bcma.co.uk
*Publishes BCMA National
Practitioner Register listing
practitioners who belong
to member organisations.*

**British Heart
Foundation**
14 Fitzhardinge Street
London W1H 6DH
Tel: 020 7935 0185
Web: www.bhf.org.uk

**British Herbal Medicine
Association (BHMA)**
Sun House
Church Street
Stroud
Gloucestershire GL5 1JL
Tel: 01453 751389
Web: www.bhma.info
*Provides an information
service and list of qualified
herbal practitioners.*

British Holistic Medical Association (BHMA)
59 Lansdowne Place
Hove BN3 1FL
Tel: 01273 725951
Web: www.bhma-sec.dircon.co.uk
For directory of members and book/tape list.

British Homeopathic Association (incorporating the Homoeopathic Trust)
15 Clerkenwell Close
London EC1R 0AA
Tel: 020 7566 7800
Web: www.trust.homeopathy.org
Provides an information service, newsletter, booklist and names of homeopathic practitioners.

BNA (British Nursing Association)
The Colonnades
Beaconsfield Place
Hatfield
Hertfordshire AL10 8YD
Tel: 01707 263544
Web: www.bnauk.com
For qualified nurses, home helps and nursing care assistants to care for people in their own homes.

British Pain Society
21 Portland Place
London W1B 1PY
Tel: 020 7631 8870
Web: www.britishpainsociety.org
An alliance of professionals advancing the understanding and management of pain for the benefit of patients.

British Red Cross
9 Grosvenor Crescent
London SW1X 7EJ
Tel: 020 7235 5454
Or look in the telephone directory for a local contact number.
Web: www.redcross.org.uk
For advice about arranging for equipment on loan.

British Society for Allergy, Environmental and Nutritional Medicine
PO Box 7
Knighton
Powys LD7 1WT
Tel: 0906 302 0010
Web: www.bsaenm.org.uk
For details of doctors who have a special interest in how diet and environmental factors are linked to chronic illness.

CancerBACUP
3 Bath Place
Rivington Street
London EC2A 3JR
Tel: 020 7696 9003
Web: www.cancerbacup.org.uk
Provides a range of services, support and publications for patients, relatives and professional workers.

Care and Repair
Castle House
Kirtley Drive
Nottingham NG7 1LD
Tel: 0115 070 9091
Advice and practical assistance for older and disabled people, and those on low incomes, to help them improve their home conditions.

Carers UK
20-25 Glasshouse Yard
London EC1A 4JS
Tel: 020 7490 8818
CarersLine:
0808 808 7777
Web: www.carersonline.org.uk
Acts as the national voice of carers, raising awareness and providing support, information and advice.

Centre for Study of Complementary Medicine
51 Bedford Place
Southampton SO15 2DT
Tel: 023 8033 4752
For advice and details of specialist organisations.

Charity Search
25 Portview Road
Avonmouth
Bristol BS11 9LD
Tel: 0117 982 4060,
9.00am-3.00pm, Monday to Thursday
Helps link older people with charities that may provide grants to individuals. Applications in writing are preferred.

Community Transport Association
Highbank
Halton Street
Hyde
Cheshire SK14 2NY
Tel: 0161 351 1475
Advice: 0161 367 8780
Services to benefit providers of transport for people with mobility problems. Also keeps a database of all Dial-a-Ride schemes.

Council for Complementary and Alternative Medicine (CCAM)
63 Jeddo Road
London W12 6HQ
Tel: 020 7724 9103
Advice and details of specialist organisations. Send an SAE for details.

Counsel and Care
Lower Ground Floor
Twyman House
16 Bonny Street
London NW1 9PG
Tel: 020 7485 1566
Web: www.
counselandcare.org.uk
Offers free counselling, information and advice for older people and carers, including specialist advice about using independent agencies and the administration of trust funds for single payments (eg respite care).

Crossroads Care
10 Regent Place
Rugby
Warwickshire CV21 2PN
Tel: 01788 573653
Web: www.crossroads.
org.uk
For a range of services, including personal and respite care.

Department of Health
Quarry House
Quarry Hill
Leeds LS2 7UE
Web: dh.gov.uk

Department for Work and Pensions
Benefit Enquiry Line:
0800 88 22 00
www.dwp.gov.uk

Depression Alliance (England)
35 Westminster Bridge Road
London SE1 7JB
Tel: 020 7633 0557
Text: 020 7928 9992
Web: www.
depressionalliance.org
Provides information, support and understanding to everyone affected by depression and campaigns to raise awareness of the illness.

Depression Alliance (Scotland)
3 Grosvenor Gardens
Edinburgh EH12 5JU
Tel: 0131 467 3050

Depression Alliance (Cymru)
11 Plas Melin
Westbourne Road
Whitchurch
Cardiff CF4 2BT
Tel: 029 2069 2891

Diabetes UK
10 Parkway
London NW1 7AA
Tel: 020 7424 1000
Web: www.diabetes.org.
uk
The national organisation for people with diabetes. Provides information and advice on a wide range of topics.

Dial-a-Ride (DART)
See Community Transport Association (page 203).

Disablement Information and Advice Lines (DIAL UK)
St Catherine's Hospital
Tickhill Road
Doncaster
South Yorkshire DN4 8QN
Tel: 01302 310123
Web: www.dialuk.org.uk
For your nearest group giving information and advice about disability.

Disability Living Allowance Unit
Customer Enquiry Unit
Swansea SA99 1BL
Tel: 0870 240 0010
Information about exemptions from road tax for vehicles used exclusively by or for disabled people.

Disability Living Centres Council
Redbank House
4 St Chads Street
Manchester M8 8QA
Tel: 0161 834 1044
Web: www.dlcc.org.uk
For the Disability Living Centre nearest you, where you can see aids and equipment.

Disabled Living Foundation
380-384 Harrow Road
London W9 2HU
Tel: 020 7289 6111
Equipment helpline: 0870 603 9177
Minicom: 0879 603 9176
Web: www.dlf.org.uk
Information and advice about all aspects of daily living (and aids) for people with disability.

Disabled Persons Railcard Office

PO Box 1YT
Newcastle upon Tyne
NE99 1YT
Helpline: 0191 269 0303
Web: www.railcard.co.uk
For railcards offering concessionary fares. An application form and useful booklet called Rail Travel for Disabled Passengers can be found at most larger stations or from the address above.

Drinkline

7th Floor, Weddell House
13-14 Smithfield
London EC1A 9DL
Tel: 020 7332 0202
National alcohol helpline that provides confidential information, help and advice about drinking to anyone, including people worried about someone else's drinking.

Expert Patients Programme

Web: www.expertpatients.
nhs.uk
A government funded initiative giving patients the opportunity to gain the knowledge, skills and confidence to manage their conditions more effectively.

EXTEND

22 Maltings Drive
Wheathampstead
Hertfordshire AL4 8QJ
Tel/Fax: 01582 832760
Provides exercise in the form of movement to music for people over 60 years and less able people of all ages.

Heart UK (formerly Family Heart Association)

7 North Road
Maidenhead
Berkshire SL6 1PE
Tel: 01628 628638
Web: www.heartuk.org.uk
Provides information about coronary heart disease and its management.

HELPBOX

The Help for Health Trust
Freepost
Winchester SO22 5BR
Tel: 01962 849100
A computer database that holds a vast and comprehensive range of health-related information.

Holiday Care Service

7th Floor, Sunley House
4 Bedford Park
Croydon
Surrey CR0 2AP
Tel: 0845 124 9971
Text: 0845 124 9976
Web: www.holidaycare.
org.uk
Information and advice on holidays, travel facilities and respite care available for people with disabilities, on low income or with special needs.

Homeopathic Medical Association

6 Livingstone Road
Gravesend
Kent DA12 5DZ
Tel: 01474 560336
(10.00am-1.00pm and
2.00pm-4.00pm, Monday
to Friday)
Web: www.the-hma.org
For the names of trained homeopathic doctors.

Hospice Information Service

St Christopher's Hospice
51-59 Lawrie Park Road
London SE26 6DZ
Tel: 0870 903 3903
(9.00am-5.00pm, Monday
to Friday)
Web: www.
hospiceinformation.info
For information about hospices and hospice care.

ICAS (Independent Complaints Advocacy Service)

For details in your area, see the relevant page on the website for the Commission for Public-Patient Involvement in Health (CPPiH).
Web: www.cppih.org/icas.
html

INPUT

Pain Management Unit
St Thomas' Hospital
London SE1 7EH
Web: www.inputpainunit.
org
For information about treatment at a residential pain management unit.

Institute of Complementary Medicine (ICM)

PO Box 194
London SE16 7QZ
Tel: 020 7237 5165
(10.00am-3.00pm,
Monday to Friday)
Web: www.icmedicine.
co.uk
Advice and details of specialist organisations.

International Federation of Professional Aromatherapists
ISPA House
82 Ashby Road
Hinckley
Leicestershire LE10 1SN
Tel: 01455 637987
Web: www.ifparoma.org
For a booklist and details of qualified practitioners in your area.

International Federation of Reflexologists
78 Edridge Road
Croydon
Surrey CR0 1EF
Tel: 020 8667 9454
For names of qualified reflexologists in your area.

International Glaucoma Association
108 Warner Road
Camberwell
London SE5 9HQ
Helpline: 020 7737 3265
Web: www.iga.org.uk
Offers support and information about glaucoma for patients and professional workers and funds research.

Institute for Optimum Nutrition
Blades Court
Deodar Road
London SW15 2NU
Tel: 020 8877 9993
Web: www.ion.ac.uk
A charity set up to study research and best practice in nutrition. Membership offers access to a newsletter, factsheets, a library and many other benefits.

Marie Curie Cancer Care
89 Albert Embankment
London SE1 7TP
Tel: 020 7599 7777
Web: www.mariecurie.
org.uk
Provides in-patient centres and runs home nursing service for day and night care.

Marie Curie for Scotland
29a Albany Street
Edinburgh EH1 3QN
Tel: 0131 456 3700
As above.

Migraine Action Group
Unit 6, Oakley Hay Lodge
Business Park
Great Folds Road
Great Oakley
Northants NN18 9AS
Helpline: 01536 461333
Web: www.migraine.org.
uk
Provides information and support for migraine sufferers, their families and friends.

Migraine Trust
45 Great Ormond Street
London WC1N 3HZ
Tel: 020 7278 2676
Web: www.migrainetrust.
org
Offers a range of services including information and advice, news, books and factsheets, research, awareness raising and educational courses. The organisation is a member of a consortium of charities called Headache UK.

Motability
Gate House, West Gate
Harlow
Essex CM20 1HR
Helpline: 01279 635666
Applications: 0845 456
566 (local call rate)
Web: www.motability.
co.uk
Advice about cars, scooters and wheelchairs for disabled people.

Motor Neurone Disease Association
PO Box 246
Northampton NN1 2PR
Helpline: 08457 626262
(9.00am-5.30pm and
7.00-10.30pm, Monday to
Friday, 10.00am-6.00pm,
Saturday and Sunday)
Web: www.
mndassociation.org
Offers care and support to sufferers and their families through a network of regional care advisers, literature, free equipment loan service and limited financial support; the organisation also funds research.

Motor Neurone Disease Advice, Care and Support (Scottish)
76 Firhill Road
Glasgow G20 7BA
Tel: 0141 945 1077
Services similar to above.

Multiple Sclerosis Society of GB and Northern Ireland
25 Effie Road
London SW6 1EE
Helplines: 020 7222 3123
(Counselling London 24Hrs)
0121 476 4229
(Counselling Midlands 10am-11.00pm)
028 9064 4914
(Counselling N Ireland 9.00am-5.00pm)
0131 226 6573
(Counselling Scotland 10.00am-11.00pm)
Offers help and support to MS sufferers and their carers.

MS Trust
Spirella Building
Bridge Road
Letchworth
Hertfordshire SG6 4ET
Tel: 01462 476700
Web: www.mstrust.org.uk
Provides specialist support and information for people with multiple sclerosis, families and professional workers; the organisation also funds research.

National Association for Colitis and Crohn's Disease
4 Beaumont House
Sutton Road
St Albans
Hertfordshire AL1 5HH
Helpline: 0845 130 3344
Web: www.nacc.org.uk
Offers advice and support to people with ulcerative colitis and Crohn's disease.

National Association of Councils for Voluntary Service
3rd Floor, Arundel Court
177 Arundel Street
Sheffield S1 2NU
Tel: 0114 278 6636
Web: www.nacvs.org.uk
Promotes and supports the work of councils for voluntary service, or look in the telephone directory for your nearest local office.

National Association for the Relief of Paget's Disease
1 Church Road
Eccles
Manchester M30 0DL
Tel: 0161 707 9225
Offers information and advice about the bone disorder Paget's disease.

National Asthma Campaign
Providence House
Providence Place
London N1 0NT
Helpline: 0845 701 0203
(9.00am-7.00pm, Monday to Friday)
Offers advice and help to asthmatics.

National College of Hypnosis and Psychotherapy
12 Cross Street
Nelson
Lancashire BB9 7EN
Tel: 01282 699378
Publishes an annual directory of practitioners.

National Endometriosis Society
Suite 50, Westminster Palace Gardens
1-7 Artillery Row
London SW1P 1RL
Helpline: 0808 808 2227
Web: www.endo.org.uk
Provides information and support for women with endometriosis, their families and friends.

National Federation of Shobmobility UK
The Hawkins Suite
Enham Place
Enham Alamein
Andover SP11 6JS
Tel: 08456 442 446
Web: www.justmobility. co.uk
An independent charity supporting shopmobility schemes.

National Federation of Spiritual Healers
Old Manor Farm Studio
Church Street
Sunbury on Thames
Middlesex TW16 6RG
Tel: 0891 616080
(premium rate line)
Advice and details of spiritual healers.

National Osteoporosis Society
Camerton
Bath BA2 0PJ
Helpline: 0845 450 0230 (10.00am-5.00pm Monday, 9.30am-5.00pm Tuesday to Friday)
Web: www.nos.org.uk
Offers information and support and works to improve the prevention, diagnosis and treatment of this fragile bone disease.

National Rheumatoid Arthritis Society
Briarwood House
11 College Avenue
Maidenhead
Berkshire SL6 6AR
Helpline: 01628 670606
(9.30-5.30 Monday to Friday)
Web: www.rheumatoid.org.uk
Provides advice and support to people with rheumatoid arthritis and their families.

Neuropathy Trust
PO Box 26
Nantwich
Cheshire CW5 5FP
Helpline: 01270 611828
(10.00am-4.00pm, Tuesday to Thursday)
Web: www.neurocentre.com
Provides information and support to people who suffer with peripheral neuropathy and neuropathic pain and to health care professionals.

New World Aurora
16a Neal's Yard
Covent Garden
London WC2H 9DP
Tel: 020 7379 5972
For catalogue of relaxation music tapes.

NHS Direct
Tel: 0845 46 47
Web: www.nhsdirect.nhs.uk
A 24-hour nurse-led helpline providing confidential health care advice and information.

NHS Smoking Helpline
Tel: 0800 169 0 169
Offers help and support to give up all forms of smoking.

Northern Ireland Office, Department for Health and Social Services
Web: www.dhsspsni.gov.uk

The Outsiders
BCM Box Outsiders
London WC1N 3XX
Tel: 020 7354 8291
Sex and Disability Helpline: 0707 499 3527
Web: www.outsiders.org.uk
A nationwide self-help community, which has recently taken over some of the roles of SPOD, including its Helpline.

No Panic
Tel: 0800 783 1531
Telephone service only for an information pack about dealing with anxiety and panic disorder. Callers are asked to leave details of their name and address on an answerphone as the organisation cannot return calls.

Pain Relief Foundation
The Clinical Sciences Centre
University Hospital Aintree
Lower Lane
Liverpool L9 7AL
Tel: 0151 529 5820
Web: www.painrelieffoundation.org.uk
Focuses on fighting pain through research, education and information – for patients, relatives and professional workers.

Pain Support UK
Web: www.painsupport.co.uk
An online resource providing information and support for those in pain, including a regular newsletter, a Confidential Contact Club, a Discussion Forum and advice about self-help techniques for reducing or controlling pain.

Parkinson's Disease Society of the UK
215 Vauxhall Bridge Road
London SW1V 1EJ
Helpline: 080 8800 0303
(9.30am-5.30pm, Monday to Friday)
Web: www.parkinsons.org.uk
Offers support and advice to people with the disease, their families and friends.

The Patients Association
PO Box 935
Harrow
Middlesex HA1 3YJ
Tel: 020 8423 9111
Helpline: 08456 084455
Web: www.patients-association.com
Provides a wide range of patient-related information, details of support groups and campaigns on behalf of patients.

Quitline
Tel: 0800 002 200
A freephone helpline that provides confidential and practical advice for people wanting to give up smoking.

RADAR (Royal Association for Disability and Rehabilitation)
12 City Forum
250 City Road
London EC1V 8AF
Tel: 020 7250 3222
Web: www.radar.org.uk
Information about aids and mobility, holidays and leisure.

Research Institute for Consumer Affairs (trading as Ricability)
30 Angel Gate
326 City Road
London EC1V 2PT
Tel: 020 7427 2460
Textphone: 020 7427 2469
Web: www.ricability.org.uk
Tests and evaluates goods and services for disabled and older people, including ordinary consumer products as well as special aids and equipment.

Royal College of Psychiatrists
12 Belgrave Square
London SW1X 8PG
Tel: 020 7235 2351
Web: www.rcpsych.ac.uk
Publishes a range of information for dealing with anxieties, phobias, depression and bereavement. Send an SAE for details.

St John Ambulance
Look in the telephone directory for local contact number.
For advice about arranging equipment on loan and first aid courses.

The Samaritans
46 Marshall Street
London W1V 1LR
Tel: 08457 90 90 90 (24 hours every day)
Text: 08457 90 91 92 (24 hours every day)
Web: www.samaritans.org.uk
Offers confidential emotional support to any person who is suicidal or despairing.

Scotland's Health on the Web
Web: ww.show.scot.nhs.uk
Online health information provided by NHS Scotland.

Sickle Cell and Thalassaemia Information Centre
Homerton Hospital
Homerton Row
London E9 6SR
Tel: 020 8510 7412/3
Offers a range of services including social and health care support, information, counselling, training and education.

Sickle Cell Society
54 Station Road
London NW10 4LU
Helpline: 020 8961 4006
Offers an information pack on sickle cell disease and trait.

Society of Homeopaths
2 Artizan Road
Northampton NN1 4HU
Tel: 01604 621400
For names of homeopathic practitioners.

Sports Council
16 Upper Woburn Place
London WC1H 0QP
Tel: 020 7263 1500
Websites:
www.sportengland.org
www.sportni.org
www.sportscotland.org.uk
www.cyngor-chwaraeon-cymru.co.uk
Provides general information about all sports. For each country, contact main office or visit the appropriate website.

Stress Management Training Institute
Foxhills
30 Victoria Avenue
Shanklin
Isle of Wight PO37 6LS
Tel: 01983 868166
Publishes a wide range of materials to help reduce stress: leaflets, audio tapes, books and newsletter.

Trigeminal Neuralgia Association UK
PO Box 413
Bromley
Kent BR2 9XS
Tel: 020 8462 9122
Web: www.tna-uk.org.uk
Offers advice and support to sufferers of this neurological condition.

Tripscope
The Vassall Centre
Gill Avenue
Bristol BS16 2QQ
Tel/Text: 08457 585641
Web: www.tripscope.org.uk
A national travel and transport information service for older and disabled people.

UK College for Complementary Health Care Studies
Wembley Centre for Health and Care
Barham House
116 Chaplin Road
Wembley HA0 4UZ
Tel: 020 8795 6656/6178
For a list of qualified practitioners of therapeutic massage.

UK Register of IBS Therapists
PO Box 57
Warrington
Cheshire WA5 1FG
Tel: 01925 629899
Web: www.ibs-register.co.uk
Provides up-to-date information on IBS including research, complementary therapy, professional papers and links to a bulletin board.

UK Reiki Federation
PO Box 1785
Andover
Hants SP11 0WB
Tel: 01264 773774
(10.30am-12.30pm, Monday to Thursday)
Web: www.reikifed.co.uk
Provides lists of practitioners and information on self-regulation and standards.

University of the Third Age (U3A)
National Office
26 Harrison Street
London WC1H 8JG
Tel: 020 7837 8838
Web: www.u3a.org.uk
Day-time study and recreational classes for older people. Send an SAE for further information, or look in the telephone directory for local branch.

Unwind Pain and Stress Management
Melrose
3 Alderlea Close
Gilesgate
Durham DH1 1DS
Tel: 0191 384 2056
Offers support to people who suffer stress due to pain. Self-help programmes, books, takes and helpline backup are available. Send an SAE for details.

Volunteer Development Agency (England)
(formerly National Association of Volunteer Bureaux)
New Oxford House
16 Waterloo Street
Birmingham B2 5UG
Tel: 0121 633 4555
Web: www.vda.org.uk
Information on matters related to volunteering, with a directory of volunteer bureaux and other publications.

Welsh Office: Ombudsman for Wales
Tel: 029 2039 4621
Web: www.ombudsman.org.uk
Provides advice on patients' rights in Wales.

Winged Fellowship
Angel House
20-32 Pentonville Road
London N1 9XD
Tel: 020 7833 2594
Web: www.wft.org.uk
Provides respite care and holidays for physically disabled people, with or without a partner.

Glossary

Acupressure points
Points situated at various places over the body where a practitioner exerts pressure to balance the flow of invisible energy running through body.

Allodynia
Extreme sensitivity to pain caused by even the lightest sensation.

Analgesic
Pain-relieving.

Articular cartilage
Specialised, fibrous connective tissue.

Atheroma
A build-up of fatty deposits inside an artery, eventually leading to a blockage.

Atherosclerosis
Degeneration of the middle coat of the arterial wall which becomes thickened due to deposits of fatty-like substances.

Balloon angioplasty
A procedure to widen the arteries by means of an inflatable balloon.

Bursa
A pouch of fibrous tissue containing synovial fluid, the fluid that normally lubricates the joints.

Bypass surgery
Surgery that allows the blood to circulate through the heart by means of vessels 'grafted' or 'transplanted' from another part of the person's own body to replace two, three or all four of the main vessels (arteries and veins) that usually perform this task. This is a major procedure, but can prevent fatal heart attacks if the vessels are damaged.

Dorsal horn
The part of the spinal cord where nerve fibres carrying sensory messages congregate (or collect or meet) before being redirected to the brain along different routes according to type, whether painful or non-painful sensations.

Double blind research trial
A method of scientific investigation often used to assess the usefulness of new medicines or treatments. Two groups of people (subjects) are given two different treatments, but even the people administering the treatment do not know which group each individual belongs to although the information is coded to be drawn upon later. The effects of the treatment on all subjects are observed so that an objective judgement can be made as to its usefulness.

Enzyme
The name given to a chemical 'ferment' produced by living cells. A small amount of the substance is capable of triggering large-scale changes in vital body functions, particularly within the digestive system.

Fallopian tubes
Tubes that are attached at one end to the uterus (womb), one on each side, with the other end lying close to the ovaries, where finger-like protrusions catch the ejected eggs.

Gate Control Theory
A theory put forward by
Professors Melzack and
Wall to describe the processes by which the sensa-
tion of pain is able to, or
can be prevented from,
registering in the brain.

Hormone
These are 'chemical
messengers' produced
in various organs around
the body, which are then
released, to be carried
by the blood to another
(sometimes distant) body
part in order to affect its
function.

Hyperalgesia
Over-sensitivity to touch.
Hyperalgesia can cause
touch that should be neu-
tral or even pleasurable to
feel actively unpleasant.

Iritis
Inflammation of the iris, the
coloured part of the eye.

Nerve fibres
Tiny 'wires' in the body
that carry messages to the
brain. Three main types
are involved with the study
of pain. These are A-delta
fibres (which carry pain
messages, quickly, to the
brain), C fibres (which
carry pain messages
rather more slowly to the
brain), and A-beta fibres
which carry pleasurable or
soothing messages and
which are the fastest of
all to act. The reason the
A-beta fibres act so fast is
that their route to the brain
is a shorter one than that
of the A-delta or C fibres.

Neuralgia
Nerve pain.

Opioid receptor
Points at which opium-
like substances, whether
produced internally by the
body or given as a drug,
can become attached.
Opium-like substances
(from whatever source)
act to suppress nerve
impulses and dampen
down the brain's percep-
tion of pain. The amount
of substance received by
the body is crucial. Small
doses of opium used
recreationally produce
excitement; medicinal-size
doses swiftly induce deep
(pain-free) sleep; poison-
ous-size doses can be
fatal.

Palpitation
A condition where the
heart beats forcibly and
sometimes irregularly so
that the person is con-
scious of its action.

Placebo effect
This term describes what
happens when a person
receives a 'dummy' or
fake treatment or medi-
cine, rather than a real,
active one. Some people
in this position do show
an improvement, either
because receiving any
treatment makes them
feel better in themselves,
or because their condition
was improving anyway.
The use of the placebo is
common in double-blind
trials, as it provides a
yardstick for measuring
the effectiveness of the

'real' treatment in the other
group. But allowances
must be made for it if the
results of any research trial
are to be accurate.

Prostaglandin
A substance originally
discovered in semen (and
then thought to arise in the
prostate gland, hence the
name). It is now known
that these substances
(in different forms) are
produced, but not stored,
by most living cells. Their
mode of action is rapid
and short acting, but precisely how they work is not
yet clear. They are known
to play a part in muscle
contraction and have an
important role in the control of pain and inflammation. For example, aspirin
relieves pain by preventing
(inhibiting) the formation of
certain prostaglandins.

**Radiofrequency
thermo-coagulation**
A technique where heat
generated by radio waves
is used to block the pain
messages that travel along
nerves.

Respiratory depression
A slow, quiet and shallow
breathing rate which may
be irregular.

Bibliography

Carr, E. and Mann, E. (2000) *Pain: Creative approaches to effective management.* Palgrave.

Gillie, O. (Out of print) *Escape from Pain.* Self-Help Direct.

Hofstadter, D. and Dennett, D.C. (1985) *The Mind's I.* Bantam.

McCaffery, M. and Beebe, A. (1994) *Pain: A clinical manual of nursing practice.* CV Mosby.

Melzack, R. and Wall, P. (1965) 'Pain mechanisms: a new theory'. *Science,* 150: 971-979.

Melzack, R. and Wall, P. (1999) *Textbook of Pain,* 4th edition. Churchill Livingstone.

Moore, A. et al. (2003) *Bandolier's Little Book of Pain.* Oxford University Press.

Wall, P. (1999) *The Science of Suffering.* Weidenfeld & Nicolson.

About Age Concern

Age Concern is the UK's largest organisation working for and with older people to enable them to make more of life. We are a federation of over 400 independent charities that share the same name, values and standards.

We believe that ageing is a normal part of life, and that later life should be fulfilling, enjoyable and productive. We enable older people by providing services and grants, researching their needs and opinions, influencing government and media, and through other innovative and dynamic projects.

Every day we provide vital services, information and support to thousands of older people of all ages and backgrounds.

Age Concern also works with many older people from disadvantaged or marginalised groups, such as those living in rural areas or black and minority ethnic elders.

Age Concern is dependent on donations, covenants and legacies.

Age Concern England
1268 London Road
London SW16 4ER
Tel: 020 8765 7200
Fax: 020 8765 7211
Website:
www.ageconcern.org.uk

Age Concern Scotland
113 Rose Street
Edinburgh EH2 3DT
Tel: 0131 220 3345
Fax: 0131 220 2779
Website:
www.ageconcernscotland.org.uk

Age Concern Cymru
Ty John Pathy
Units 13 and 14 Neptune Court
Vanguard Way
Cardiff CF24 5PJ
Tel: 029 2043 1555
Fax: 029 2047 1418
Website: www.accymru.org.uk

Age Concern Northern Ireland
3 Lower Crescent
Belfast BT7 1NR
Tel: 028 9024 5729
Fax: 028 9023 5497
Website: www.ageconcernni.org

Publications from Age Concern Books

Better Health in Retirement *Dr Anne Roberts*

A little attention to your body's changing needs and some knowledge of how to deal with common illnesses can lead to a long and healthy retirement. Written in non-medical language, Dr Anne Roberts gives practical, expert advice and information to help everyone keep as healthy as possible in later life. Topics include:

- developing a healthy lifestyle

- health checks and screening

- common illnesses of later life

- using the Health Service

- help for older carers

This book also provides clear guidance on areas such as depression, sleeping well and relaxation techniques. Positive and upbeat, this book will equip readers with all of the information needed to take charge of their own health.

£6.99   ISBN: 0-86242-251-5

Know Your Complementary Therapies *Eileen Inge Herzberg*

People who practise natural medicine have many different ideas and philosophies, but they all share a common basic belief: that we can all heal ourselves – we just need a little help from time to time.

Written in clear, jargon-free language, the book covers an introduction to complementary therapies, including acupuncture, herbal medicine, aromatherapy, spiritual healing, homeopathy and osteopathy. Uniquely focusing on complementary therapies and older people, the book helps readers to decide which therapies are best suited to their needs, and where to go for help.

£9.99   ISBN: 0-86242-309-0

Age Concern Books' titles by Toni Battison

Caring for someone with depression
£6.99 0-86242-389-9

Caring for someone with cancer
£6.99 0-86242-382-1

Caring for someone with a heart problem
£6.99 0-86242-371-6

Caring for someone with memory loss
£6.99 0-86242-358-9

To order from Age Concern Books

Call our **hotline: 0870 44 22 120** (for orders or a free books catalogue)
Opening hours 9am–7pm Monday to Friday, 10am–5pm Saturday and Sunday

Books can also be ordered from our secure online bookshop: **www.ageconcern.org.uk/shop**

Alternatively, you can write to Age Concern Books, Units 5 and 6 Industrial Estate, Brecon, Powys LD3 8LA. Fax: 0870 8000 100. Please enclose a cheque or money order for the appropriate amount plus p&p made payable to Age Concern England. Credit card orders can be made on the order hotline.

Our **postage and packing** costs are as follows: mainland UK and Northern Ireland: £1.99 for the first book, 75p for each additional book up to a maximum of £7.50. For customers ordering from outside the mainland UK and NI: credit card payment only; please telephone for international postage rates or email sales@ageconcernbooks.co.uk

---

Bulk order discounts

Age Concern Books is pleased to offer a discount on orders totalling 50 or more copies of the same title. For details, please contact Age Concern Books on 0870 44 22 120.

Customised editions

Age Concern Books is pleased to offer a free 'customisation' service for anyone wishing to purchase 500 or more copies of most titles. This gives you the option to have a unique front cover design featuring your organisation's logo and corporate colours, or adding your logo to the current cover design. You can also insert an additional four pages of text for a small additional fee. Existing clients include many prominent names in British industry, retailing and finance, the trade union movement, educational establishments, public, private and voluntary sectors, and welfare associations. For full details, please contact Sue Henning, Age Concern Books, Astral House, 1268 London Road, London SW16 4ER. Fax: 020 8765 7211. Email: hennins@ace.org.uk

Information Line/Factsheets subscription

Age Concern produces 50 comprehensive factsheets designed to answer many of the questions older people (or those advising them) may have. These include money and benefits, health, community care, leisure and education, and housing. For up to five free factsheets, telephone 0800 00 99 66 (8am–7pm, seven days a week, every week of the year). Alternatively you may prefer to write to Age Concern, FREEPOST (SWB 30375), ASHBURTON, Devon TQ13 7ZZ.

For professionals working with older people, the factsheets are available on an annual subscription service, which includes updates throughout the year. For further details and costs of the subscription, please contact Age Concern at the above Freepost address.

We hope that this publication has been useful to you. If so, we would very much like to hear from you. Alternatively, if you feel that we could add or change anything, then please write and tell us, using the following Freepost address: Age Concern, FREEPOST CN1794, London SW16 4BR.

Index

A-beta fibres 18, 163
A-delta fibres 17–18
abscesses 36, 37, 56, 57, 119–20
aching muscles 20
Across Trust 198
Action on Pain 10
acupressure 131, 157–58
acupuncture 12, 131, 154, 158
acute pain 35, 36–37, 117
Addenbrooke's Hospital, Cambridge:
    Pain Clinic 97, 100, 113
addiction to drugs 128–29
adhesions 43–44
'adjuvant' therapy 125
advocacy services 115
age: and pain 10
aids and equipment 135, 136
air travel 197–98
alcohol consumption 187–89
allodynia 19, 75
alternative therapies 154, 155
amitriptyline 126
amputees 24–25, 39, 137
anaesthetics, long-acting 133–34
analgesics 125
analogue pain scales 109, 112
angina 15, 38, 44–46, 50, 65, 123, 189,
    190, 191
ankylosing spondylitis 50
anti-convulsant drugs 125
antidepressants 39, 113, 125–26
anti-spasmodic drugs 126
anxiety 15, 44, 63, 87, 143, 146, 149,
    185
arms, massaging 166–67
aromatherapy 131, 141, 154, 158–60
arteriograms 95
arthralgia 46
arthritis 21–22, 27–28, 31, 37, 38, 46–47,
    116, 118, 126
ankylosing spondylitis 50
    osteoarthritis 47–48, 63
    polyarthritis 49, 55

psoriatic 49–50
reactive 50
rheumatoid 48–49
Arthritis Care 131
arthroscopies 93
aspirin 80, 124
assessment, pain 97–98, 115
    in-patient monitoring 103
    and information provided by patient
    98, 101–102
    of levels of pain 102
    with laminated pain charts 103–106
    physical examinations 103
asthma 50–51, 157
atherosclerosis 44, 72, 189
attitudes to pain 85–87
auto-suggestion 28–29
Ayurvedic remedies 12, 171

Bach Flower Remedies 160–62
back pain 24, 31, 38, 51–54, 58, 70,
    179–80
    treatments 51, 52, 157, 162
    see also arthritis; lumbago; osteoporo-
    sis; sciatica
badminton 182
balloon angioplasty 45–46
barium enemas 94
barium meals 94
baths, scented 160
behavioural responses 22–23
Bell's palsy 54
benzodiazepines 127
biofeedback 171
biopsies 92
bladder stones 73
blood tests 91–92
Blue Badge Scheme 195
bones
    fractured 20, 38, 69, 145, 199-200
    metastasis 43
    and osteomyelitis 70
    and osteoporosis 70–71

painful 20
books and leaflets, useful 33–34, 113
boredom: and stress 146
bowls, playing 181
brain, role of the 17
breathing techniques 149–50, 151, 152
Brief Pain Inventories 106–108
bronchoscopies 93
Brufen 124

C fibres 17, 18
cancer 38, 41–43
    and blood tests 92
    treatments 40, 126, 136
cannabis 127, 192
carpal tunnel syndrome 49, 54–55
central post-stroke pain (CPSP) 78
cerebral palsy 55, 75
cerebral-vascular accidents (CVAs) 77–78
chemical actions 19
chemotherapy drugs 126
chest pains 24
chiropractic 52, 130, 171
cholecystitis 36, 59
cholecystograms 95
chronic bowel disease 79
chronic pain 31, 35, 37–38, 117
Clinical Nurse Specialists (CNSs) 100
clinics, pain 99–101
CNSs see Clinical Nurse Specialists
coach trips 197
codeine 124
cognitive behavioural therapy 24, 130–31
cold therapy 136, 137
colic/colicky pain 20, 63, 126
colitic arthritis 50
collagen diseases 55, 72, 139
colonoscopies 93
colour therapy 155
Community Transport Association 196
Community Transport schemes 195
complaints, making 115
complementary therapies 12, 35, 131,
    141, 154–57, 173
computed tomography (CT) scans 95–96
consciousness: and pain 12–13
constipation 56
    from drugs 128
counselling 131–32, 149, 154, 199

CPSP see central post-stroke pain
cramps, leg 182; see peripheral vascular
    disease
Crohn's disease 56
cryotherapy 133
CT see computed tomography
cultural background: and pain 85
CVAs see cerebral-vascular accidents
cycling 181
cystoscopies 93
cytotoxic drugs 126

dancing 182
dental problems 56–57
dependence, drug 129
depression 63, 117, 122, 143, 145,
    157, 185–87
    and alcohol 187–88
    see also Hospital Anxiety Depression
Descartes, René 11
diabetic neuropathy 57
diagnosing pain 89
Dial-a-Ride 195
diaries, keeping
    pain 112, 113
    stress 145–46
diarrhoea 56, 63, 143
diazepam 127
diet(s)
    build-up 176–77
    healthy 174–75
    and sleeping problems 184
    specialist advice on 177–78
Disability Living Allowance Unit 196
distraction 132
diverticulitis 57
doctor, going to your 89–90
drugs 12, 19, 32, 121, 122, 124, 199
    addiction to 127, 128–29
    and alcohol 188–89
    anti-convulsant 125
    antidepressant (tricyclics) 125–26
    anti-spasmodic 126
    cannabis 127, 192
    chemotherapy/cytotoxic 126
    and clinical trials 27
    containers 121–22
    dependence on 129
    methods for taking 122–24

for mild pain 124
for moderate pain 124-5
over-the-counter 128
for phantom pain 39
sedative 125
for severe pain 125
and side effects 128
steroid 90, 127
tolerance to 129
see also specific illnesses
duodenal ulcers 81–82, 86
duodenoscopies 93
dyspepsia/indigestion 20, 57–58, 143

ears, pain in 20
eating problems 143, 175–76
see also diet(s)
electrolytes 91
emotional sensitivity: and pain 85–86
endogenous opioids 19
endometriosis 58
endorphins 158
equipment see aids and equipment
essential oils 159-60
exercise 178–80, 199
leisure activities and sports 181–82
and safety precautions 180–81
and sleeping problems 185
Expert Patients Programme 132–33
EXTEND 182
eyes, pain in 14, 20, 60–61

families, effects on 23, 29, 117–18
fatigue 68, 161, 185
Fentanyl 123
fibreoptic endoscopies 92–93
fibrin tissue 44
fibromyalgia 58
forehead massage 165
freezing therapy see cryotherapy
'frozen' shoulder 59

gall stones 20, 59–60
gardening 183–84
gastric ulcers see stomach ulcers
gastroscopies 93
Gate Control Theory (Melzack and Wall)
11, 12, 15-16, 16, 17, 18, 87
glaucoma 14, 60–61
glucosamine 28

golf 181
golfers' elbow 59
gout 61

HAD see Hospital Anxiety Depression
haemoglobin levels 91
haemorrhoids 62
headaches 15, 65, 134, 143, 157, 158;
see also meningitis; migraines
heat therapy 133, 136, 137
helplines 149
herbal medicine 128, 154, 155–56; see
also Bach Flower Remedies
hernias 39, 62–63
hiatus hernia 62
hip degeneration 39, 47, 63
holidays 196–98
homeopathy 128, 154, 162–63
hormone replacement therapy (HRT)
70–71
Hospital Anxiety Depression (HAD) questionnaires 109, 110–11
Hospital Car Schemes 195
HRT see hormone replacement therapy
hydrotherapy 171
hyperalgesia 19
hypermobility syndrome 139–40
hypnosis/hypnotherapy 12, 131, 171

IASP see International Association for the
Study of Pain
IBS see irritable bowel syndrome
ibuprofen 124
ileitis 56
imipramine 126
impotence 194
indigestion 20, 57–58, 143
infections 36, 37, 40, 43
inflammation 36
inhalation 160
injections
intrasmuscular 123
intravenous 123
subcutaneous 123–24
INPUT 138–39
insomnia see sleeping problems
intermittent claudication 72
International Association for the Study
of Pain (IASP) 25, 35, 38
Internet websites 32–33, 119

intramuscular injections 123
intravenous injections 123
intravenous urograms 94
iridology 155
irritability 142, 143, 146, 147
irritable bowel syndrome (IBS) 20, 63–64
ischaemia 64–65
IVPs see intravenous urograms

kidney function tests 92
kidney stones 20, 36, 73–74

laminated pain charts 103–106
leaflets see books and leaflets
leg cramps 182; see peripheral vascular
    disease
leg ulcers 72, 82
liver function tests 92
long-acting anaesthetics 133-34
lumbago 65
lymphograms 95

McGill Pain Questionnaire (MPQ) 109
magnetic resonance imaging (MRI) scans
    95, 96
mammograms 95
massage 12, 131, 155, 163–67
    aromatherapy 141, 160
    see also Shiatsu
mastectomies 39
mattresses, special 135
ME see myalgic encephalomyelitis
Medical Patient Transport Schemes 195
medication see drugs
meningitis 68
migraines 15, 65–67, 116, 117, 144, 157
Migraleve 66,140
minerals 177
monitoring pain 98
    in-patient 103
    out-patient 106–12
morphine 124, 125
    side effects 125, 128
    suppositories 123
Motability 195
motor neurone disease 67
mouth, the
    absorption of drugs in 123
    ulcers 79-80

MRI see magnetic resonance imaging
    scans
multiple sclerosis (MS) 67–68, 127
muscle-relaxants 127
muscles, aching 20
muscular tension 134, 135
    massage for 165
music therapy 167
myalgia 68
myalgic encephalomyelitis (ME) 68
naloxone 27
National Back Pain Association 131
nausea 25, 157
neck, the
    injuries and pain 68; see also whiplash
    massaging 166
nerve blocks 133
nervous system, role of the 17-19
neuralgia 20, 69
    postherpetic 75–76
    trigeminal 23, 69, 125
neurofibroma 69
neurofibromatosis 69
neurotransmitters 87, 126
NHS Direct Online 32
night-time: and pain 86
non-steroidal anti-inflammatory drugs
    (NSAIDs) 32, 48, 124, 125, 126
    side effects 48, 49, 126–27, 128
noradrenaline 87
nortriptyline 126
NSAIDs see non-steroidal anti-inflamma-
    tory drugs
nuclear medicine 96
Nurofen 125

occupational therapists (OTs) 101
oesophagoscopies 93
oils, essential 159–60
opioids 12, 32, 125
    endogenous 19, 27
osteoarthritis 47–48, 63, 134, see
    also arthritis
osteomyelitis 70
osteopathy 52, 130, 134, 171
osteoporosis 70–71
OTs see occupational therapists

Paget's disease 71
pain 9–15, 31–32

and the brain and nervous system 17–19
diagnosing and reporting 89–90; see also assessment, pain
diversity of 20
psychological aspects of 23–25, 28–29, 40
reactions to 22–23, 85–88
types of 35–40
see also Gate Control Theory
pain control/relief 40–41
    barriers to 113–14
    non-drug techniques 130–38
    see drugs
pain management units 138–39
pain modulation theory 19
Pain Relief Foundation 83–84
painful arc syndrome 59
painkillers see drugs
PALS (Patient Advice and Liaison Services) 115
pancreatitis 82
paracetamol 124
parking concessions 195
Parkinsonism 71–72
Parkinson's disease 71
patches, self-adhesive (painkillers) 123
Patients Association 84
periarthritis 59
peripheral vascular disease 65, 72, 182, 190, 194
peritonitis 44, 56, 81
Perthes' disease 47
phantom pain 24–25, 39, 137
pharmacists 101, 128
PHN see postherpetic neuralgia
physiotherapists/physiotherapy 52, 101, 134, 163
piles 62
pithiatism 29
placebo effect 25–27, 28
pleurisy 44, 49
polyarthritis 49, 55
polymyalgia rheumatica 72
postherpetic neuralgia (PHN) 75–76
posture and position 135
prostaglandins 19, 80
psoriatic arthritis 49–50
psychological aspects of pain 23–25, 28–29, 40; see also placebo effect

psychologists, clinical 101
psychosomatic pain 40
psychotherapists/psychotherapy 101, 130–31; see also counselling
pyelograms see intravenous urograms
pyloric stenosis 81

Qi Gong 172
questionnaires, out-patient 106–12

RADAR 198
radioactive isotope scans 96
radiotherapy 136
rail fares, concessionary 195
Raynaud's syndrome 72–73
referred pain 39, 43, 58, 59
reflexology 154, 167–69
Reiki 168
relaxation techniques 132, 145, 149–53
renal colic 73–74
repetitive strain injury (RSI) 74
rheumatism 74
rheumatoid arthritis 48–49
RSI see repetitive strain injury

Samaritans 149
scans 95
    computed tomography (CT) 95–96
    magnetic resonance imaging (MRI) 96
    radioactive isotope 96
    ultrasound/ultrasonic 97
scar damage 43
sciatica 31, 75
scoliosis 75
secondary pain 40
sedative drugs 125
self-help support networks 149, 199
self-help treatments 118–20, 200
self-hypnosis 131
self-massage 164
septicaemia 117
serotonin 87
sexual relationships 192–94
Shiatsu 171
shingles 69, 75
Shopmobility schemes 196
shoulders
    'frozen' 59
    massaging 166
    referred pain in 58, 59

stiffness in 72
sickle cell disease 76, 91
sigmoidoscopies 93
skin creams, pain-killing 127
sleeping problems/insomnia 143, 144, 147, 152, 184–85
'slipped' discs 27, 51–52, 65, 69, 75
smoking 70, 73, 145, 189–91, 192; see also cannabis
solpadol 53, 124
somatic pain 40
spastic colon see irritable bowel syndrome
spinal cord, taking drugs via 123
spinal stenosis 30
spondylosis 76
sports 181, 182
steroid drugs 90, 127
'stitch' 20
stomach ulcers 20, 58, 80–81
stomatitis 80
stress 44, 79, 131, 141–42, 172
    causes and triggers 142, 143–45, 146
    and diary-keeping 145–46
    finding support 148–49
    management of 145
    and self-help 146–48
    warning signs and symptoms 143
strokes 65, 77–78
subcutaneous injections 123–24
support groups 83–84
suppositories 123
surgery
    and post-operative pain 87
    removal of nerves 133
swimming 181
syringomyelia 17, 78
systemic lupus 55
systemic sclerosis 55

T'ai-chi Ch'uan 172
'talking' therapies see counselling
Taxicard services 196
telephone helplines 149
temperature: and pain relief 136–37
tendinitis 78
tendons 38; see tendinitis; tenosynovitis
tennis elbow 59
tenosynovitis 74, 78

TENS (Transcutaneous Electrical Nerve Stimulator) machines 137–38
testosterone 194
tests
    biopsies 92
    blood 91–92
    fibreoptic endoscopies 93–94
    see also scans; X-rays
therapists, qualified 156–57
TIAs see transient ischaemic attacks
tiredness 68, 144, 161, 185
tolerance, drug 129
tranquillisers 127
transient ischaemic attacks (TIAs) 77
transport schemes 194–96
travel sickness 157
treatments see pain control/relief
tricyclic drugs 113, 125–26
trigeminal neuralgia 23, 69, 125
Tripscope 196
tumours 20, 38, 40; see cancer

ulcers 79, 82
    duodenal 81–82, 86
    gastric see ulcers, stomach
    mouth 79–80
    stomach 20, 56, 58, 80–81, 126
    varicose (leg) 72, 82
ultrasound (ultrasonic) scans 97
urea 92
ureter stones 73

Valium 127
vaporisation 159–60
varicose (leg) ulcers 72, 82
venograms 95
Viagra 194
visceral pain 40
visual body charts 109
visual charts see laminated pain charts
visualisation 132, 170–71
vitamins 177

walking (for exercise) 181
'wheat bags' 137
wheelchairs 195, 197
whiplash 82–83
Wilde, Oscar: De Profundis 13
Winged Fellowship 198
wryneck 83

X-rays 93
    arteriograms 95
    barium enemas 94
    barium meals 94
    cholecystograms 95
    intravenous urograms 94
    lymphograms 95
    mammograms 95
    venograms 95

yoga 12, 154, 182